W0071670

The Nutrition of Goats

Agricultural and Food Research Council
(Now incorporated in the Biotechnology and Biological Sciences
Research Council)
Technical Committee on Responses to Nutrients
Report no. 10

Reprinted from
Nutrition Abstracts and Reviews
Series B
Volume 67 No. 11

CAB INTERNATIONAL

CABI Publishing is a division of CAB International

CABI Publishing
CAB International
Wallingford
Oxon OX10 8DE
UK

Tel: +44 (0)1491 832111
Fax: +44 (0)1491 833508
Email: cabi@cabi.org
Web site: www.cabi-publishing.org

CABI Publishing
44 Brattle Street
4th Floor
Cambridge, MA 02138
USA

Tel: +1 617 395 4056
Fax: +1 617 354 6875
Email: cabi-nao@cabi.org

A catalogue record for this book is available from the British Library, London, UK

ISBN 0 85199 216 1

First published 1998
Transferred to print on demand 2004

Printed and bound in the UK by Antony Rowe Limited, Eastbourne.

Contents

List of Tables

Preface

The Working Party on the Nutrition of Goats was established in 1987 by the former AFRC Technical Committee for Responses to Nutrients (TCORN) with the Terms of Reference set out on p. xv. At that time there were no formal recommendations on the nutrient requirements of goats in the UK, although various small leaflets had appeared, based largely on overseas recommendations. The Working Party rapidly concluded that recommendations for UK goat producers should be closely related to the then existing UK recommendations for the nutrient requirements of cattle and sheep (ARC 1980, 1984). To achieve this aim, a thorough survey of all relevant information relating to goat nutrition in temperate zones would be required, requiring more time than had originally been envisaged. During this extended period of activity by the Working Party, revisions of the nutrient recommendations for cattle and sheep were published for energy, (AFRC 1990), protein (AFRC 1992), minerals (AFRC 1991) and energy and protein (AFRC 1993), necessitating further review and revision of the recommendations for goats. Extensive technical editing of the manuscript was undertaken by Dr B.A. Stark in 1991. In 1993 Mr G. Alderman joined the Working Party to review its recommendations in the light of the more recent AFRC reports, particularly those for energy and protein incorporated in AFRC (1993). The present report is the outcome of these various efforts.

Despite these problems, we believe that we have achieved the aims originally set out and have provided a completely new set of recommendations for the nutrient requirements of goats in terms compatible with the current AFRC recommendations for cattle and sheep.

Nutrition Abstracts and Reviews (Series B)
AGRICULTURAL AND FOOD RESEARCH COUNCIL
(Now incorporated in the Biotechnology
and Biological Sciences Research Council)
Technical Committee on Responses to Nutrients.
Report Number 10. Nutrition of Goats
This report was prepared by an AFRC Working Party
on the Nutrition of Goats

Membership

Chairman Dr J.D. Sutton, Institute of Grassland and Environmental
Research, Hurley. (a)

Members Mr A. Mowlem, Goat Advisory Bureau, Reading. (b)
Dr E. Owen, Department of Agriculture, University of
Reading. (a)
Dr A.J.F. Russel, Macaulay Land Use Research Institute,
Penicuik. (c)
Dr R.H. Smith, formerly National Institute for Research in
Dairying, Shinfield.[1]
Dr B.A. Stark, Nutrition Consultant, High Wycombe. (d)
Dr T.T. Treacher, Institute of Grassland and Environmental
Research, Hurley. (e)
Dr J.M. Wilkinson, Chalcombe Agricultural Resources,
Hurley. (f)
Mr G. Alderman, Department of Agriculture, University of
Reading.[2]

Notes: [1]Deceased.
[2]From 1993 onwards only.

Current addresses:
(a) Department of Agriculture, University of Reading, Earley
Gate, Reading RG6 6AT.
(b) Water Farm, Stogursey, Bridgewater, Somerset TA5 1PS.
(c) Newton Bank, Frankscroft, Peebles EH45 9DX.
(d) Cap House, Llangua, Abergavenny, Gwent NP7 8HD.
(e) Dpto. de Produción Animal, ETSIAM, Universidad de
Córdoba, 14080 Córdoba, Spain.
(f) Department of Animal Physiology & Nutrition, The
University, Leeds LS2 9JT.

Terms of reference

1. To review current information on the energy, protein, major mineral, trace element and vitamin requirements for growth and lactation.
2. To provide information in a suitable form to improve feeding standards for productive goats.
3. To identify areas of ignorance requiring further research and to make recommendations for such.

Terminology and Symbols Used

This glossary of terms, symbols and units is identical to that adopted in AFRC (1993) for the sake of uniformity and ease of cross reference between the two publications. The principles used in the construction of the glossary were:

UPPERCASE LETTERS are used for **energy and nutrient supply** (per animal) per day, either **g/d** or **MJ/d** as appropriate.
The same symbols, enclosed in square brackets, e.g. **[DUP]**, are used for **concentrations, g/kg or MJ/kg**, except where existing usage dictates otherwise.
Lower case letters are used for rates, efficiencies and proportions, which are either expressed as decimals (not percentages), or with relevant units, e.g. g/MJ.

The units and abbreviations used for weight, time etc., are as in the SI system. Crude protein (CP) or (P) is taken as $6.25 \times$ Nitrogen (N), except for milk where it is taken as $6.38 \times N$

Subscripts are used to differentiate between metabolic functions as follows:

b   Basal metabolism
c   Concepta/gravid uterus/pregnancy
d   Dermal losses, scurf and hair
f   Live weight gain
g   Gain/loss in live weight in lactating animals
l   Lactation
m   Maintenance
n   Nitrogen utilisation, combined with the above set
p   Production
t   Time in days
w   Fibre growth

A	Activity allowance, J/kg/ml or kJ/kg daily
AA	Amino acids
a	Proportion of water soluble N in the total N of a feed
[ADIN]	Acid detergent insoluble nitrogen in a feed, g/kg DM
B	Derived parameter to predict energy retention
b	Proportion of potentially degradable N other than water soluble N in the total N of a feed
BEN	Basal endogenous nitrogen, $g/kgW^{0.75}$ daily
[BF]	Butterfat content of milk, g/kg
c	Fractional rumen degradation rate per hour of the *b* fraction of feed N with time, t
C_L	Plane of nutrition correction factor in calculating ME requirements of lactating ruminants
CP, [CP]	Crude protein, g/d in a diet or g/kg DM in a feed
DE, [DE]	Digestible energy, MJ/d of a diet or MJ/kg DM in a feed
dg	Extent of degradation of feed nitrogen (or CP) at time, t
DMI, [DM]	Dry matter, intake, kg/d, or content, g/kg in a feed
DMTP	Digestible microbial true protein, g/d, ie truly absorbed in the intestines (= metabolisable protein from microbes)
[DMTP]/[MTP]	True absorbability of amino acids from microbial true protein
DOM, [DOMD]	Digestible organic matter, kg/d in a diet or g/kg DM in a feed
DOMR	Apparently digestible organic matter that is apparently digested in the rumen, kg/d in a diet or g/kg DM in a feed
DUP, [DUP]	Digestible undegraded protein (N × 6.25), the amount or proportion of undegraded feed protein that is truly absorbed, g/d in a diet or g/kg DM in a feed
E, [E]	Net energy, MJ/d or g/kg DM
E_c	Net energy retained in concepta, MJ/d
E_f	Net energy retained in growing animal, MJ/d
E_g	Net energy retained or lost in weight change in lactating ruminants, MJ/d
E_l	Net energy secreted as milk, MJ/d
E_m	Net energy for maintenance, MJ/d
E_{mp}	Net energy for maintenance and production, MJ/d
E_t	Net energy content of concepta at time t, MJ
E_w	Net energy retained as goat fibre, MJ/d
EBW	Empty-body weight, kg
ERDN, [ERDN]	Effective rumen degradable nitrogen, which has the potential to be captured by rumen microbes at a rumen digesta outflow rate of r/hour
ERDP, [ERDP]	Effective rumen degradable protein (ERDN × 6.25)
$[EV_g]$	Energy value of tissue lost or gained, MJ/kg
$[EV_l]$	Energy value of milk, MJ/kg
F	Fasting metabolism, $MJ/(kg\ fasted\ weight)^{0.67}$ daily.
FOM, [FOM]	Fermentable organic matter, g/d or g/kg DM of a feed
F_p, F%	Proportion of forage in the diet dry matter (or as percent)
FI	Milk fat intake by kids, g/d
FME, [FME]	Fermentable ME of a diet, MJ/d or MJ/kg DM in a feed
GE, [GE]	Gross energy of a diet, MJ/d or MJ/kg DM in a feed

I	Intake of dietary ME, MJ/d scaled by fasting metabolism, F
k	Derived parameter to predict energy retention
k_{aai}	Efficiency with which a mixture of absorbed amino acids in ideal proportions is used for the net synthesis of protein as tissue, fibre or milk
k_c	Efficiency of utilisation of ME for growth of the concepta
k_f	Efficiency of utilisation of ME for weight gain
k_g	Efficiency of utilisation of ME for weight change when lactating
k_l	Efficiency of utilisation of ME for milk production
k_m	Efficiency of utilisation of ME for maintenance
k_t	Efficiency of utilisation of mobilised tissue for lactation
k_n	Net efficiency of utilisation of absorbed amino acids, = 1 for maintenance and = $k_{aai} \times$ RV for other purposes
k_{nb}	Efficiency for basal metabolism (BEN)
k_{nc}	Efficiency for growth of concepta (pregnancy)
k_{nd}	Efficiency for synthesis of scurf and hair
k_{nf}	Efficiency for growth
k_{ng}	Efficiency for gain when lactating
k_{nl}	Efficiency for lactation
k_{nm}	Efficiency for maintenance
k_{nw}	Efficiency for fibre growth
L	Level of feeding as a multiple of MJ of ME for maintenance
[La]	Lactose content of milk, g/kg
LWG (or W)	Live weight gain or change, both either ± g/d or kg/d
M_c	ME requirement for growth of concepta, MJ/d
M_f	ME requirement for live weight gain, MJ/d
M_g	ME requirement for live weight change when lactating, MJ/d
M_l	ME requirement for milk production, MJ/d
M_m	ME requirement for maintenance, MJ/d
M_{mp}	ME requirement for maintenance and production, MJ/d
M_w	ME requirement for fibre growth, MJ/d
MCP, [MCP]	Microbial crude protein supply, g/d or g/kg DM
M/D	Metabolisable energy, MJ/kg DM of a diet; see also [ME] for a feed or diet
ME, [ME]	Metabolisable energy, MJ/d or MJ/kg DM of a feed or diet; see also M/D for a diet
ME_{fat}	Metabolisable energy from fat (oil) in a feed, MJ/kg DM
ME_{ferm}	Metabolisable energy from fermentation acids in fermented or ensiled feed, MJ/kg DM
MER	Metabolisable energy requirement, MJ/d
MFN, [MFN]	Metabolic faecal nitrogen, g/d or g/kg DM of a diet
MN, [MN]	Microbial nitrogen, g/d, g/kg DOMR or g/MJ FME
MP, [MP]	Metabolisable protein, g/d from a diet or g/kg DM of a feed
MP_c	MP requirement for growth of concepta, g/d
MP_f	MP requirement for live weight gain, g/d
MP_g	MP requirement for live weight gain when lactating, g/d
MP_l	MP requirement for milk production, g/d
MP_m	MP requirement for maintenance, g/d

MP_w	MP requirement for fibre growth, g/d
MPR	Metabolisable protein requirement, g/d
[MTP]/[MCP]	Proportion of microbial crude protein present as true protein
n	Lactation week number
NAN	Non-ammonia nitrogen, g/d
NP_b	Net protein equivalent of basal endogenous nitrogen (BEN), g/d
NP_c	Net protein for growth of concepta (pregnancy), g/d
NP_d	Net protein for scurf and hair growth, g/d
NP_f	Net protein accreted in gain, g/d
NP_g	Net protein accreted or mobilised when lactating, g/d
NP_l	Net protein secreted in milk, g/d
NP_m	Net protein for maintenance, g/d
NP_w	Net protein for fibre growth, g/d
NPN, [NPN]	Non-protein nitrogen, g/d of a diet or g/kg in a feed
[OMD]	Organic matter digestibility, g/kg of a diet or feed
[P]	Crude protein content of milk, g/kg
p	Effective degradability of feed N at rumen digesta fractional outflow rate, r
q_m	Metabolisability of [GE] at maintenance, [ME]/[GE]
QDN, [QDN]	Quickly degradable nitrogen, g/d of a diet or g/kg DM in a feed
QDP, [QDP]	Quickly degradable protein (QDN × 6.25), g/d or g/kg DM in a feed
QDP/MCP	Limiting efficiency of conversion of QDP to MCP
R	Energy retention (Ef), MJ/d, scaled by fasting metabolism (F)
r	Rumen digesta fractional outflow rate per hour
RDP, [RDP]	Rumen degradable protein (N × 6.25), g/d in a diet or g/kg DM in a feed, for a given rumen digesta fractional outflow rate, r
RV	Relative value of the amino acid mixture supplied, compared with the ideal amino acid mixture
SDN, [SDN]	Slowly degradable nitrogen, g/d or g/kg DM in a feed, for a given rumen digesta fractional outflow rate, r
SDP, [SDP]	Slowly degradable protein (SDN × 6.25)
SDP/MCP	Limiting efficiency of conversion of SDP to MCP
[SNF]	Solids not fat in milk, g/kg
TDMI	Total dry matter intake of a diet, kg/head per d
TEN	Total endogenous nitrogen, g $N/kgW^{0.75}$ per d
TP, [TP]	Tissue protein (ARC 1980) = net protein, (NP) g/d or [NP], g/kg
UDN, [UDN]	Undegradable dietary nitrogen, g/d of a diet or g/kgDM in a feed, for a given rumen digesta fractional outflow rate, r
UDP, [UDP]	Undegradable dietary protein (UDN × 6.25), g/d of a diet or g/kgDM in a feed
UEN	Urinary endogenous nitrogen, g $N/kgW^{0.75}$ daily
W	Live weight of the animal, kg
W_m	Mature body weight of the animal, kg
W (or LWG)	Live weight gain or change, both either ± g/d or kg/d
Y	Yield of milk, kg/d
y	Microbial protein yield in the rumen, g MCP/MJ of FME

1. Introduction

1.1 The goat industry

The long history of the goat as a domesticated animal in the UK is dominated by its use on small holdings for milk production. Until recently almost all herds were very small and great attention was placed on the individual animal and its performance. As a result of dedicated breeding, the best animals are now capable of producing 1500 to 2000 kg of milk per year (Mowlem 1988). Average yields of milk on larger holdings approach 1000 kg per head from adult animals.

Recently, interest in goat production has increased in Europe, especially in France. In the UK a similar expansion has occurred, both on agricultural holdings (Wilkinson and Stark 1987b) and on small holdings (Islay and Jura Goat Society 1985). Until 1985 much of this expansion was in milk production, and it was estimated that the population of goats in British dairy herds in 1991 was about 90,000. The principal breeds contributing to the total are British Saanen (21%), British Toggenburg (14%), Anglo-Nubian (12%), Saanen (7%), British (5%), British Alpine (5%) and Toggenburg (4%) (Islay and Jura Goat Society 1985).

Production in the UK of the two major types of goat fibre, mohair and cashmere, is of very recent origin and the introduction in 1981 of Angora goats from New Zealand and Tasmania created a minor revolution in the goat industry. More animals were imported from Texas a few years later. By coincidence, work on cashmere production, based originally on feral goats and later on crosses with imported stock brought in as live animals, embryos and semen, began at the same time. Although the UK output of both types of fibre is still very small, the economic straits of many traditional forms of animal production have made a number of livestock producers seek alternative enterprises, and the number of fibre-producing goats, particularly cashmere goats, increased rapidly. Through the extensive use of embryo transfer initially, the number of Angora and Angora cross goats in Britain increased from a few dozen in 1984 to around 10,000 in 1992 (Mowlem *pers comm*). The number of cashmere goats also increased rapidly and was estimated to be about 10,000 in 1992 (Russel *pers comm*).

Alongside the increased population of goats has come a greater interest in larger-scale goat farming. Dairy herds in excess of 100 animals are now well-established and managed along similar lines, using similar expertise, to dairy cow herds. Herds of goats developed for fibre production are managed by farmers accustomed to keeping large sheep flocks.

1.2   Goat products

The main products from the goat comprise milk, meat and fibre.

1.2.1   Milk

Goats' milk has a similar gross composition to that of cows' milk, although there are differences within the fat fraction, with a higher proportion of small fat globules in goats' milk. For this reason goats' milk is recommended for babies and other people who may be experiencing difficulty in digesting cows' milk.

Cheese from goats' milk is comparable to that from cows' milk, but goats' milk forms a softer curd and as a result goat cheeses tend to be softer than cheeses from cows' milk. Goats' milk butter and cream are both white and thus noticeably different in appearance to comparable cows' milk products.

1.2.2   Meat

The most striking characteristic of goat meat is the different distribution of fat compared to that in sheep meat. Goat meat has a very low proportion of intermuscular fat and at similar carcase weights goats may be expected to produce carcases with a lower proportion of subcutaneous and intramuscular carcase fat and a higher proportion of non-carcase fat in the abdominal cavity compared to sheep. This lower proportion of carcase fat is reflected in a higher proportion of bone in the carcase of goats.

Dairy goats, in particular, have longer legs and longer bodies than sheep, and from the point of view of those accustomed to dealing with lambs, their conformation as meat animals is poor. Consequently goat carcases tend to be undervalued, and the development of a goat meat industry in Britain has been less rapid than that of the dairy and fibre industries.

1.2.3 Fibre

Mohair is used mainly in knitwear and, to a lesser extent, in apparel cloth and soft furnishings. Mohair fibres have a much smoother surface than wool, which makes spinning more difficult and causes loops of single fibres to appear on the surface of the yarn. This property is often made a feature; loops are deliberately introduced and the final product brushed to give the typical "halo" effect characteristic of mohair garments. It is also frequently manufactured in blends with synthetic fibres. Mohair is subject to the vagaries of fashion and consequently prices fluctuate markedly.

Cashmere is much finer than either wool or mohair and, weight for weight, has a substantially higher insulating value. The finest cashmere is used in the manufacture of very high quality knitwear, while the slightly coarser fibres are woven into cloth. Cashmere is regarded as the most luxurious of animal fibres. World markets are under-supplied and prices are consequently higher and relatively more stable than for wool and mohair.

Goat skins, and particularly skins from kids, are a source of very high quality leather sought after for book-binding, drum skins and gloves.

1.3 The need for information on the nutrition of the goat

Although the majority of goats are still kept in small herds, the lack of research and extension work on goats in the UK is in sharp contrast to that in other countries, especially France, the USA and Scandinavia. The goat has been used extensively as a model for the cow in physiological research but, in contrast, sheep rather than goats have been used as models in nutrition research. Thus the developing British goat industry faces a dearth of relevant scientific and technical support, particularly with respect to nutrition. The Agricultural and Food Research Council's Technical Committee on Responses to Nutrients (AFRC TCORN) therefore commissioned this review on the current state of knowledge with respect to the nutrition of the goat, particularly in the UK.

Several countries have produced recommendations on goat nutrition but the basis of the recommendations is usually obscure, and many are simply repetitions or minor revisions of others published elsewhere. Relatively few scientific papers have been written and many of the published studies are not relevant to conditions in the UK being, for example, conducted under tropical or sub-tropical conditions. Most feed intake research has been carried out in France where maize silage and lucerne are often fed, but these feeds are uncommon for goats in the UK.

In preparing this report, particular efforts have been made to locate original sources. The general approach in the Agricultural Research Council's published recommendations, The Nutrient Requirements of Ruminant

Livestock (ARC 1980), has been followed and, where appropriate, reference has also been made to the reports of Working Parties which have subsequently examined the ARC (1980) recommendations. In particular, consideration has been given to Supplement No.1 to the Nutrient Requirements of Ruminant Livestock (ARC 1984), to TCORN Report No. 9, the Nutrient Requirements of Ruminant Animals: Protein (AFRC 1992) and to the AFRC Advisory Manual on the Energy and Protein Requirements of Ruminants (AFRC 1993). TCORN Report No. 6, A Reappraisal of the Calcium and Phosphorus Requirements of Sheep and Cattle (AFRC 1991) has also been taken into consideration. Where the information on goats is adequate it has been compared with that for cattle and sheep. In other instances, requirements are based on those for ruminants in general, and the need for more information specific to the goat has been noted.

This report comprises a review of information on the composition of the goat and its products; feed intake and digestive physiology; energy, protein, mineral and vitamin nutrition of the goat; and production responses to changes in nutrient supply. Recommendations are made for further research as appropriate.

2. Composition of Products

2.1 Body and carcase

Estimations of nutrient requirements using the factorial method as in ARC (1980) necessitate accurate knowledge of patterns of deposition of tissue during the growth of kids and of patterns of change in tissues during weight increase or mobilisation of body reserves in various stages of the productive cycle in the adult female. For dairy goat production in the UK, this information is needed for the British Saanen breed, which is predominant in commercial goat keeping. In the long term it would be desirable to have information for the other main breeds to see if they differ radically from the British Saanen. Unfortunately, there are few data on growing kids and none of real value for the adult. Thus, the nutrient requirements for British dairy goats, particularly lactating females, calculated in this publication will have a limited precision until sound data are obtained on the composition of weight changes in goats.

2.1.1   Kids at birth

Three references were found to the composition of male kids slaughtered 48 hours after birth (Table 2.1). Jagusch *et al* (1983) reported the composition of 10 Saanen kids with a mean live weight of 4.27 kg and Sanz Sampelayo *et al* (1990) reported the composition of 6 Granadina kids with a mean empty body weight (EBW) of 2.11 kg. The composition of these two groups of kids differed considerably, which may have been due to differences in breed but could also have been affected by methods of processing or analysis. More recent results for 8 two-day-old British Saanen kids (Yan *et al* 1993) are very similar to those of Jagusch *et al* (1983). The Working Party used the following mean values from these experiments: 25 g fat, 170 g crude protein and 5.0 MJ energy/kg EBW.

There are no published data on the mineral content of kids at birth, and it is suggested that values for new born lambs should be used. ARC (1980)

Table 2.1: Composition of empty body of kids at 2 days of age.

Breed type:	Saanen		Granadina Sanz Sampelayo et al (1990)
Authors:	Jagusch *et al* (1983)	Yan *et al* (1993)	
Live-weight (kg)	4.27	3.88	–
Empty body weight (EBW, kg)	3.99	3.64	2.11
Fat (g/kg EBW)	24.3	22.7	29.4
Protein (g/kg EBW)	189.8	177.2	144.3
Energy (MJ/kg EBW)[1]	5.43	5.07	4.58

[1] Calculated using (ARC 1980) energy values of 39.3 MJ/kg fat and 23.6 MJ/kg protein.

gives the following values (g/kg EBW) for new born lambs weighing 4 kg: ash 40.0, calcium (Ca) 13.0, phosphorus (P) 7.0, magnesium (Mg) 0.45, potassium (K) 1.8 and sodium (Na) 2.4.

2.1.2   Growing kids

(a)   Pre-weaning

The papers by Jagusch *et al* (1983) and Sanz Sampelayo *et al* (1990) included the composition of kids given milk or milk substitutes in the first 3 to 4 weeks of life. At a similar EBW the contents of fat and protein of the kids (Table 2.2) differed very radically between the two sets of data. The energy contents were, however, more similar, with little difference between the kids from the experiment of Jagusch *et al* (1983) and the restricted group from the work of Sanz Sampelayo *et al* (1990).

Table 2.2: Composition of empty body of kids reared on milk or milk substitute and slaughtered at approximately one month of age.

Feeding level	Jagusch *et al* (1983)	Sanz Sampelayo *et al* (1990)	
	Grazing on range	*Ad libitum*	80% of *ad lib*
Age at slaughter (days)	21	30	30
Empty body weight (EBW, kg)	5.63	5.98	4.32
Fat (g/kg EBW)	65.4	105	80.3
Protein (g/kg EBW)	181.9	145.4	151.2
Energy (MJ/kg EBW)[1]	6.86	7.56	6.72

[1] Calculated using (ARC 1980) energy values of 39.3 MJ/kg fat and 23.6 MJ/kg protein.

Sanz Sampelayo *et al* (1990) also reported the composition of kids slaughtered at 15 days of age; they had lower fat contents (79 g/kg EBW on *ad libitum* feeding and 57 g/kg EBW on 80% of *ad libitum*) than the 30-day-old kids, and their composition was similar to the Saanen kids of Jagusch *et al* (1983) slaughtered at 21 days of age. The protein content of 144 g/kg EBW for both levels of intake was very similar to that of the kids slaughtered at birth and at 30 days. In the same experiment, contents of fat and energy were strongly correlated with EBW and were not affected by feeding level or whether goats' milk or milk substitute was fed.

The depositions of fat, crude protein and energy in each unit of EBW gain, from the composition of kids slaughtered at two days of age and at 3 or 4 weeks of age (Table 2.3), showed similarity between the data for the two breeds, and the means of the values from the two experiments are proposed as values for the composition of weight gains in kids given goats' milk or milk substitute in the first month of life. These values are 150 g fat, 160 g protein and 9.67 MJ energy/kg EBW gain.

Table 2.3: Composition of empty body weight (EBW) gains in kids given milk or milk substitute in the first month of life.

	Jagusch *et al* (1983)	Sanz Sampelayo *et al* (1990)[1]	Mean
Period (days)	2 to 21	2 to 30	–
Fat (g/kg EBW gain)	161	138	150
Protein (g/kg EBW gain)	165	152	160
Energy (MJ/kg EBW gain)[2]	10.22	9.01	9.67

[1] Mean of 4 treatments.
[2] Calculated using (ARC 1980) energy values of 39.3 MJ/kg fat and 23.6 MJ/kg protein.

As discussed in Section 7.1, it appears more appropriate in the absence of specific information to consider the mineral composition of live-weight gain in the goat to be similar to that of cattle rather than sheep. The Ca and P contents of live-weight gain are considered in more detail, in relation to requirements, in Section 7. Based on ARC (1980) values for cattle, the contents of the other major minerals in the EBW gain of kids (g/kg) are: Mg 0.45, K 2.0, Na 1.5 and chlorine (Cl) 1.0. There is little reliable information on the trace element content of body tissues for cattle, sheep or goats. As fat contains virtually no minerals it is expected that, as with cattle and sheep, the mineral content of the tissues of goats will vary with body fat content, although quantitative data are not available.

The Nutrition of Goats

(b) Post-weaning

Two sets of data were found relating to the body composition of weaned, castrate males from breeds found in the UK or similar to them. Australian studies by Panaretto provided data on the composition of Saanens and Toggenburgs, which were probably of British origin. Panaretto and Till (1963) reported individual data for 13 Saanen and Toggenburg mature, castrate males ranging in live weight from 10.4 to 28.8 kg, but they did not identify the breed of individual animals. Panaretto (1963) gave the body composition of 3 Toggenburg and 7 Saanen goats ranging in weight from 9.7 to 39.6 kg. The second group of data was for 34 British Saanen castrate kids slaughtered at 21, 29, 37 and 45 kg live weight in an experiment briefly reported by Treacher *et al* (1987).

Linear and curvilinear regressions were fitted to these two sets of data. Although, in general, curvilinear relationships did not result in improvements in the accounted variance, the linear regression equations often had large negative constants. It was decided, therefore, that a model in which the intercept was forced through the origin was biologically more sound. This procedure resulted in a significantly greater amount of variance being accounted for by curvilinear regressions and in non-significant differences between the regressions fitted to the two groups of data. The common regressions are presented in Table 2.4.

Table 2.4: Regression equations fitted through zero for the body composition of Saanen/ Toggenburg-type castrate male kids in relation to live weight (W), empty body weight (EBW) and derived equations for the composition of live-weight gain.[1]

		Variance accounted for (%)
Live weight (kg) basis		
Fat (kg)	$= 0.0325\,W + 0.004291\,W^2$	89.3
Protein (kg)	$= 0.15722\,W - 0.000347\,W^2$	96.7
Energy (MJ)	$= 4.972\,W + 0.1637\,W^2$	93.6
Empty body weight (kg) basis		
Fat (kg)	$= 0.0791\,EBW + 0.004137\,EBW^2$	91.0
Protein (kg)	$= 0.20239\,EBW - 0.001173\,EBW^2$	96.1
Energy (MJ)	$= 7.894\,EBW + 0.1382\,EBW^2$	94.8
Composition of live-weight gain		
Fat (g/kg)	$= 3.25 + 8.58\,W$	–
Protein (g/kg)	$= 157.22 - 0.694\,W$	–
Energy (MJ/kg)	$= 4.972 + 0.3274\,W$	–

[1] Derived from Panaretto (1963), Panaretto and Till (1963) and Treacher *et al* (1987 and unpublished data).

(c) Cashmere and feral cross kids

The regressions in Table 2.4 have been compared with data on the body composition of cashmere and feral-cross kids from Australia and New Zealand. Ash and Norton (1987b) reported the composition of 54 cashmere kids slaughtered at approximately 10 kg EBW or 20 kg EBW after being fed on different diets. The cashmere kids had similar protein weights (Table 2.5) to the Saanen/Toggenburg type kids used to generate the regressions in Table 2.4, but the fat weight was considerably lower in the cashmere male kids than in the castrate male Saanen kids. The cashmere females, however, had a similar weight of fat at 10 kg and a much higher weight of fat at 20 kg compared to the castrate male Saanen kids.

Table 2.5: Comparison of the protein and fat content of the empty body weight (EBW) of male (M) and female (F) cashmere kids slaughtered at approximately 10 or 20 kg EBW from Ash and Norton (1987b) and of Saanen/Toggenburg-type castrate male (CM) kids of the same empty body weight calculated from regressions in Table 2.4.

Breed	Sex	EBW (kg)	Protein (kg)	Fat (kg)	Energy (MJ)[1]
Cashmere	M	10.01	1.81	0.56	64.7
Saanen	CM	10.01	1.91	1.21	92.9
Cashmere	F	9.61	1.62	0.97	76.4
Saanen	CM	9.61	1.84	1.14	88.6
Cashmere	M	19.02	3.33	2.33	170.2
Saanen	CM	19.02	3.43	3.00	200.1
Cashmere	F	20.6	3.35	4.18	295.9
Saanen	CM	20.6	3.67	3.39	221.2

[1] Calculated using (ARC 1980) energy values of 39.3 MJ/kg fat and 23.6 MJ/kg protein.

A comparison of the above data on Saanen kids with data of Alam *et al* (1991) on Anglo-Nubian × feral and Angora × feral castrate male kids (Table 2.6) indicated similar weights of protein and fat at a fasted live weight of approximately 14 kg, although exact comparisons could not be made as fasted weights were not available for the Saanen kids. The body composition of pure Angora goats warrants further research as Treacher *et al* (1987) showed that carcases of Angora × Saanen castrate male kids slaughtered at 30 and 37 kg live weight had 27 and 37% more fat, and 56 and 84% more subcutaneous fat than the carcases of Saanen kids slaughtered at the same weights.

Table 2.6: Comparison of the composition of Anglo-Nubian × feral and Angora × feral castrate male kids (Alam *et al* 1991) with Saanen/Toggenburg-type castrate male kids from Table 2.4.

	Feral cross	Saanen
Live weight	13.8[1]	13.8[2]
Protein (kg)	2.06	2.10
Fat (kg)	1.31	1.27
Energy (MJ)	104.6	99.8

[1] Fasted live weight.
[2] Unfasted live weight.

2.1.3   Adult females

Only one reference, by Brown and Taylor (1986), was found relating to the body composition of adult females; they reported the mean composition of a heterogenous group of 15 French Alpine, Nubian and Toggenburg females ranging in live weight from 38.0 to 70.1 kg, and from 2 to 5 years of age, including both lactating and pregnant animals. Mean data for this group were: 49.3 kg EBW, 12.1 kg fat, 7.9 kg protein and 662 MJ energy.

However, it seems unlikely that this heterogenous group provides a reliable estimate of the composition of typical dairy goats. There is a clear need for measurements of the body composition of dairy goats of defined breeds, ages and stages of lactation.

2.1.4   Live-weight change in lactating goats

The live weight of goats has been observed to fall by up to about 6 kg during the first 6 to 12 weeks after parturition. As in dairy cows and ewes, the extent of weight loss varies widely and is affected by many factors, particularly the level of energy intake both preceding and following parturition. Research on lactating ewes by Cowan *et al* (1979, 1980, 1981) showed that a single value for the energy contributed to milk production by live-weight loss is of little value as losses in body fat are often accompanied by increases in gut and body water. Interpretation of weight changes is therefore confused by variations in gut fill but there is strong evidence that true tissue mobilisation of fat and probably protein occurs. Based on studies of adipose tissue metabolism by Chilliard (1985) and Morand-Fehr *et al* (1987), INRA (1988) suggested that goats lose about 1 kg live weight/week for the first month post-partum and 0.5 kg/week for a further month. Dunshea *et al* (1990) reported almost no live-weight loss in multiparous Saanen goats, whilst Badamana *et al* (1990) found that the live weight of British Saanen goats fell by about 1 kg/week in the first 4 weeks of lactation, but then remained fairly constant for the next

12 weeks. However, all sources agree that mobilisation of body reserves of fat and protein occurs in the early stages of lactation in goats, even if they cannot be strictly related to the amount of live-weight change.

2.1.4.1   Energy value of live-weight changes

There are no direct estimates of the energy values of live-weight gain and loss in lactating goats. French workers have published estimates of the net energy (NE) for milk production available from the mobilisation of body reserves and of the energy cost of the deposition of reserves, which have been derived by calculations from feeding trials, either alone or accompanied by analysis of blood non-esterified fatty acid levels and precursors of long-chain fatty acids in the diet. These calculations necessitated a considerable number of assumptions. The amounts of net energy available for milk production from 1 kg live-weight loss were calculated to be 3.7 unites fourrages lait (UFL)/kg (Morand-Fehr *et al* 1987). Since 1 UFL is defined as 1700 kcal (or 7.11 MJ) of net energy for lactation, this estimate is equivalent to approximately 26.3 MJ/kg of weight loss corrected for gut fill by subtracting 3.7 × DM intake (Sauvant and Morand-Fehr 1991).

Dunshea *et al* (1990) reported almost no live-weight loss in multiparous Saanen lactating goats but, using isotope techniques, estimated that between days 10 and 38 of lactation, the goats lost 0.1 kg live weight, 0.9 kg EBW and 1.63 kg body fat, whilst gaining 0.12 kg protein. This is equivalent to an average mobilisation of only 0.41 kg adipose tissue/week, compared to 1 kg/week found by Morand-Fehr *et al* (1987). The calculated losses in body energy were 61.2 MJ in total, equivalent to 68.0 MJ/kg loss in EBW and 612 MJ/kg of live-weight loss, with the latter clearly being unacceptable as a general value. The value of 68 MJ/kg loss in EBW is similar to the energy content of weight loss in the ewes in Cowan's experiments, which ranged from 17 to 68 MJ/kg (Cowan *et al* 1979). The daily loss of body energy (E_g) in the experiment of Dunshea *et al* (1990) was 2.2 MJ/d, identical to that proposed by INRA (1988) for the second month of lactation. Goat body composition is closer to that of cattle than sheep, so that the estimates of Gibb *et al* (1993) on the mean net energy content of live-weight losses in Friesian cows of 19.0 MJ/kg are relevant to these considerations.

Dunshea *et al* (1990) also reported that between days 38 and 76 of lactation, goats made small gains in weight, fat and protein: 0.8 kg live weight, 0.6 kg EBW, 0.42 kg fat and 0.08 kg protein. These give a gain in energy of 18.4 MJ and estimates for [EV_g] of 23.0 MJ/kg live-weight gain and 30.6 MJ/kg EBW gain, close to the estimate of 23.9 MJ/kg live-weight change of ARC (1980) for cattle and sheep. INRA (1988) allow for 1.2 kg gain/month from the fourth month of lactation in multiparous goats, for which an allowance of 0.16 UFL/d (1.14 MJ of NE/d) is made. This is equivalent to an [EV_g] of 28.4 MJ/kg.

The Nutrition of Goats

The Working Party agreed to adopt the ARC (1980) value of 23.9 MJ/kg live-weight change in lactating cattle and sheep as appropriate for nominal live-weight losses and gains in lactating goats, which can be used to estimate the energy contribution from body reserves in goats.

2.1.4.2   Net Protein content of live-weight changes

INRA (1988) state that goats have a relatively low capacity for mobilising and storing nitrogen reserves. According to Brun-Bellut *et al* (1984) protein as well as fat can be mobilised in goats in early lactation. They measured average losses of 55 g N during weeks 2 and 3 of lactation (3.9 g N/d, 24.4 g NP_g/d) in multiparous Alpine goats in negative energy balance. However, Dunshea *et al* (1990) measured a net tissue N retention of 0.7 g N/d (4.4 g NP_g/d) during days 10 to 38 of lactation when their goats were mobilising body adipose tissue while maintaining live weight. These results are not necessarily in conflict with those of Brun-Bellut *et al* (1984), which refer to days 8 to 21 of lactation, so that the net gain in protein that Dunshea *et al* (1990) recorded over days 10 to 38 may have missed recording a net loss in the first 21 days of the lactation. More evidence is needed about protein mobilisation in dairy goats in early lactation, but in the light of the higher N balance figures of Dunshea *et al* (1990), we provisionally recommend adoption of the ARC (1980) [NP_g] value for cattle and sheep of 138 g/kg. For a nominal live-weight loss of 1.0 kg per week (140 g/d) this implies a daily contribution of 20 g NP_g from live-weight loss.

To meet the protein requirements for live-weight gain in dairy goats, INRA (1988) recommended the addition of 4 g protein truly digested in the intestine (PDI)/d (0.64 g truly absorbed AA-N) for an average live-weight gain of 1.2 kg/month for multiparous goats and 13 g/d of PDI (2.1 g truly absorbed AA-N) for primiparous goats to allow for growth of 2.2 kg/month. Expressed as net protein requirements (NP_g) these are equivalent to 2.4 g NP_g/d for multiparous goats and 7.8 g NP_g/d for primiparous goats. These recommendations (taking the efficiency of AA utilisation for gain (k_{ng}) as 0.60 as in INRA 1988) imply [NP_g] values for live-weight gain of about 60 and 107 g/kg for multiparous and primiparous goats respectively. From the experiment of Dunshea *et al* (1990), a value of 100 g NP_g/kg live-weight gain can be calculated for multiparous goats. The ARC (1980) recommendation for the composition of live-weight gain is 138 g NP_g/kg for lactating cattle and 83 g NP_g/kg for sheep. Clearly, there is a need for further information on the protein composition of live-weight gain in lactating goats. In the meantime the Working Party agreed to accept the INRA (1988) recommendations.

2.1.5 *Depositions of fat, protein and energy in the gravid uterus during pregnancy*

There is no published information on the patterns of development or the composition of foetuses, the placenta, placental fluids and the uterus of goats during pregnancy. The choice was made, therefore, to follow in this report the precedent of the French standards (Morand-Fehr *et al* 1987, INRA 1988) and to base calculations of the deposition of fat, protein and energy during pregnancy in goats on the patterns of deposition in pregnant sheep. This appears to be justified as the length of pregnancy (147 days) is very similar in both species and the total weight of young at birth is also similar in goats and sheep producing two offspring, namely 108 g kid/kg doe for British Saanen goats (Treacher and Cook *pers comm*) and 127 g lamb/kg ewe (Robinson *et al* 1977). Depositions of fat, protein and energy during pregnancy in goats have been calculated using the following procedure:

1. In the absence of published data on the birth weights of kids from British breeds, birth weights have been calculated for dairy type goat kids from the mean birth weights of twin (3.95 kg) and triplet (3.65 kg) kids produced by the British Saanen herd at the former AFRC Institute of Grassland and Environmental Research (IGER), Shinfield, in 1989 (Treacher *pers comm*). A mean weight for a single kid of 4.44 kg was calculated using the ratio of single to twin lamb birth weights. For the kids of goats producing fibre, the mean weights of single or twin kids produced by the cashmere × feral herd at the Macaulay Land Use Research Institute (MLURI), Edinburgh were 2.75 and 2.25 kg respectively (Russel *pers comm*).

2. The relationships for ewes in Table 2 of Robinson *et al* (1977) were used to calculate the weights of foetuses, the placenta, foetal fluids and the empty uterus at the end of pregnancy, and at 2, 4, 6, 8, 10 and 12 weeks before parturition for goats of both breed types producing singles, twins and triplets (dairy breeds only). The adjustment of $0.5s^2$ (where s is the standard deviation of the data) recommended by those authors was used, before converting ln (w) values back to live weight (w) in kg. This study was used as the basis of the calculation because it contained a very detailed analysis of the changes in the uterus and its contents for the full range of litter sizes derived from slaughtering Finn-Dorset ewes. This information was not included among the sources to predict the gains in pregnancy in ARC (1980).

3. From the calculated weights of the various components of the gravid uterus, the depositions of fat, protein and energy were calculated for the same time intervals before kidding, using the equations relating the weight of fat and protein deposited to time from conception in days, in each foetus, the placenta, foetal fluids and empty uterus for ewes given in McDonald *et al* (1979), Tables 2 and 5. These calculated values for fat and protein deposition in the component parts of the gravid uterus were then summed. The deposition of net energy (E_c)

was calculated from the depositions of fat and protein by using the respective energy values of 39.3 and 23.6 MJ/kg specified by ARC (1980).

The calculated total depositions of fat, protein and energy during the last three months of pregnancy in the gravid uterus for goats of both breed types with different numbers of kids are shown in Table 2.8. In the earlier part of pregnancy (less than 60 days pregnant) the growth in the gravid uterus is small and can be ignored in calculations of nutrient requirements.

No information has been reported on the composition of the gravid uterus or the foetuses of goats to compare with the compositions for sheep at each point in time reported by McDonald *et al* (1979). If the figures in Table 2.6 are, in fact, representative of the composition of the kid at birth, they would result in the total energy content of twin kid foetuses being approximately 23% higher than the value derived from sheep. It was not felt that these limited values for the composition of kids at 48 hours after birth could be used to adjust the sheep values in the absence of data for goat foetuses at different stages of pregnancy. Similarly it was not felt acceptable to use figures for calves and cattle foetuses as the ratio of birth weight to maternal weight at parturition in cows, which generally produce a single calf, is 64 g/kg, about half the values for sheep and goats (127 and 108 g/kg).

4. In order to calculate the daily depositions of protein and energy required for the estimation of the daily energy and protein requirements of pregnant goats given in Table 2.8, the Gompertz and other equations given by McDonald *et al* (1979), in their Table 2, have to be differentiated. These differential equations are not given in their paper, but were derived by Neal (*pers comm*). The differentiated Gompertz equations have the form:

$$dy/dt \ (g/d) = \{a*exp(-bt) - c(f-3)\}W_p*f*10^3$$

where t   = time in days since conception
f   = number of foetuses
W_p = weight of protein per foetus, kg at time t
or W_f = weight of fat per foetus, kg at time t

The appropriate values of the constants a, b and c to be used in this set of Gompertz equations are given in Table 2.7.

Foetal fluids were found by McDonald *et al* (1979) to contain negligible amounts of fat, but an equation for the accumulation of protein in foetal fluids was given in their Table 5. The amount of daily gain in protein in foetal fluids is calculated as the product of that equation and the relevant third degree polynomial for weight of foetal fluids given by Robinson *et al* (1977), Table 2. When converted from kg to g and differentiated, this equation becomes:

Table 2.7: Coefficients for the differentiated Gompertz functions used to predict the daily gains in fat and protein in the individual foetus and placenta in pregnant goats.

Equations have the form:	Values of coefficients		
dy/dt (g/d) = {a*exp($-bt$) $-$ c(f$-$3)}W$_p$*f*10^3	**a**	**b**	**c**
Foetus			
Daily deposition of fat/foetus	0.364	0.0182	0.00111
Daily deposition of protein/foetus	0.326	0.0176	0.00089
Placenta			
Daily deposition of fat	4.778	0.0666	0.00109
Daily deposition of protein	2.284	0.0557	0.00096

Note: Estimated values for each foetus, the placenta, foetal fluids and empty uterus (see text) have to be summed to give total values for the gravid uterus. The ARC (1980) conversion factors are then used to convert weights of fat and protein to net energy (E_c) values.

$$dy/dt \ (g/d) = 0.075W_{fl} + (0.075t + 3.25)(0.326 - 0.00632t - 0.0000306t^2)W_{fl}$$

where W_{fl} = weight (kg) of foetal fluids at time t in days from conception.

The empty uterus was found by McDonald *et al* (1979) not to vary significantly in fat and protein content, with mean protein and fat concentrations of 134 g/kg and 23.4 g/kg respectively, so that the equation for the weight of the empty uterus from Robinson *et al* (1977), Table 2, can also be differentiated to give the daily gain in weight of the empty uterus, and hence the gains of fat and protein:

$$dy/dt \ (g/d) = 134u\{0.014193exp(-0.0038t)\} \quad \text{for protein and}$$
$$= 23.4u\{0.014193exp(-0.0038t)\} \quad \text{for fat}$$

where u is the weight (kg) of the empty uterus at time t in days.

2.2   Milk

2.2.1   Major fractions

As with the milk of dairy cows, the composition of goats' milk varies widely due to many factors including breed, stage of lactation and diet. Detailed reviews of goats' milk composition have been written by Parkash and Jenness (1968) and Jenness (1980), based on world-wide literature. The only published review of the composition of goats' milk in the UK appears to be

Table 2.8: Estimated gains in fat, protein and energy in the gravid uterus in fibre-producing goats with 1 or 2 foetuses and in dairy goats with 1, 2 or 3 foetuses.

| | Breed type | Number of foetuses | Days pregnant (weeks before parturition) | | | | | | |
			63 (12)	77 (10)	91 (8)	105 (6)	119 (4)	133 (2)	147 (0)
Total gain of:									
Fat (g)	Fibre	1	11	15	20	29	42	60	82
	Fibre	2	13	18	26	38	57	83	115
	Dairy	1	15	21	31	46	70	103	145
	Dairy	2	19	28	43	69	108	163	230
	Dairy	3	22	35	56	90	143	215	301
Protein (g)	Fibre	1	70	98	138	198	287	408	566
	Fibre	2	86	128	190	282	419	606	850
	Dairy	1	93	137	200	299	445	646	902
	Dairy	2	121	192	297	465	714	1053	1482
	Dairy	3	149	247	395	624	963	1420	1991
Energy (MJ)	Fibre	1	2.1	2.9	4.1	5.8	8.4	12.0	16.6
	Fibre	2	2.5	3.7	5.5	8.2	12.1	17.6	24.6
	Dairy	1	2.8	4.1	5.9	8.9	13.3	19.3	27.0
	Dairy	2	3.6	5.6	8.8	13.7	21.1	31.3	44.0
	Dairy	3	4.4	7.2	11.5	18.3	28.4	42.0	58.8
Daily deposition of:									
Protein (NP_c, g)	Fibre	1	1.7	2.4	3.5	5.2	7.5	9.9	12.8
	Fibre	2	2.5	3.6	5.3	8.1	11.5	15.2	19.9
	Dairy	1	2.5	3.7	5.6	8.6	12.4	16.3	20.4
	Dairy	2	4.1	6.1	9.4	14.6	21.0	27.4	34.1
	Dairy	3	5.7	8.5	13.0	20.0	28.4	36.7	45.3
Energy (E_c, MJ)	Fibre	1	0.05	0.07	0.10	0.15	0.22	0.29	0.37
	Fibre	2	0.07	0.10	0.15	0.23	0.33	0.44	0.57
	Dairy	1	0.07	0.11	0.17	0.26	0.37	0.49	0.61
	Dairy	2	0.12	0.18	0.28	0.43	0.63	0.82	1.01
	Dairy	3	0.17	0.25	0.38	0.59	0.85	1.09	1.33

that of Knowles and Watkin (1938). The results were based on samples taken at various stages of lactation from 345 goats from 8 breeds, and in addition milk yields were reported, apparently based on 10-year records of the British Goat Society.

More recently, samples of goats' milk taken throughout lactation have been analysed by the Milk Marketing Board (MMB) for England and Wales. Milk yields and compositional values for 549 goats from 7 breeds for 1986/87 are available (Morant *pers comm*), and are given in Table 2.9. The concentrations of the principal solids constituents are very similar to those in cows' milk, although the concentration of lactose in goats' milk is a little

Table 2.9: Total lactation milk yields and milk composition for dairy goats in England and Wales (Morant *pers comm*).

Breed[1]	Lactation milk yield (kg)	Composition (g/kg)			Energy value[2] [EV₁] (MJ/kg)	Net protein[3] [NP₁] (g/kg)
		Fat	Protein	Lactose		
Anglo-Nubian (116)	681	46.5	35.5	43.4	3.33	32.0
Saanen (53)	904	35.1	28.8	44.8	2.77	25.9
British Saanen (227)	970	37.6	29.2	42.8	2.84	26.3
Toggenburg (41)	672	37.1	28.6	45.8	2.87	25.7
British Toggenburg (96)	1090	37.3	29.6	43.8	2.86	26.6
British Alpine (36)	953	41.1	31.1	43.3	3.03	28.0
Golden Guernsey (25)	820	41.9	31.7	43.3	3.07	28.5

[1] Total number of lactations given in parentheses.
[2] Calculated using equation of Tyrrell and Reid (1965).
[3] Taking true (net) protein as 0.9 of crude protein.

lower, as was also noted by Parkash and Jenness (1968).

It is noteworthy that milk yields were on average about 20% lower, milk fat concentration 4.7 g/kg lower, milk protein concentration 2.8 g/kg lower and lactose concentration 2.9 g/kg higher in the results for goats sampled in 1986/87 (Morant *pers comm*) than in those for the same breeds sampled 50 years earlier (Knowles and Watkin 1938).

According to Russel and Adkins (1990) the composition of the milk of feral goats differs markedly from that of domestic goats. Results, for weeks 3 to 10 of lactation only, are given in Table 2.10. No reports of the composition of the milk of Angora goats have been located.

Table 2.10: Comparison of the yield and composition of feral[1], feral cross[2], and domestic[3] goats in weeks 3 to 10 of lactation (Russel and Adkins 1990).

Type of goat	Milk yield (kg/d)	Composition (g/kg)		Energy value,[4] [EV₁] (MJ/kg)	Net protein,[5] [NP₁] (g/kg)
		Fat	Protein		
Feral	1.27	70	34	4.30	31
Feral × domestic	1.90	49	35	3.51	31
Domestic	2.99	31	26	2.64	23

[1] Ten feral goats.
[2] Nine feral × Toggenburg and one feral × Saanen.
[3] Eight Toggenburgs and two Saanens.
[4] Calculated using equation of Tyrrell and Reid (1965).
[5] Taking true (net) protein as 0.9 of crude protein.

On the basis of the results in Table 2.9, it is suggested that for most purposes the majority of dairy goats in the UK can be divided into two main groups with respect to the concentration of the principal solids constituents. These are Anglo-Nubians, which constitute about 12% of total goats, and a group consisting of Saanens, British Saanens, Toggenburgs and British Toggenburgs (Saanen/Toggenburgs) which together constitute about 46% of total goats (Islay and Jura Goat Society 1985). Other breeds each constitute about 5% or less of the total. The mean values are given in Table 2.11.

Table 2.11: Mean composition and energy content of the milk of the two main groups of dairy goats in the UK.

Group	Composition (g/kg)			Energy value,[1] $[EV_1]$ (MJ/kg)	Net protein,[2] $[NP_1]$ (g/kg)
	Fat	Protein	Lactose		
Anglo-Nubian	47	36	43	3.355	32.4
Saanen/Toggenburg	37	29	44	2.835	26.1

[1] Calculated according to Tyrrell and Reid (1965).
[2] Taking true (net) protein as 0.9 of crude protein.

The concentrations of the major fractions are affected by other factors, including stage of lactation, level of production and parity. According to limited results by Knowles and Watkin (1938), the concentrations of butterfat [BF] and solids-not-fat [SNF] fall after parturition to a minimum at about the fourth month of lactation and increase slowly thereafter, although [BF] may reach a plateau at about the eighth month. Badamana *et al* (1990) found that in British Saanens, BF and SNF concentrations fell from about 55 and 90 g/kg respectively in week 1 of lactation to about 30 and 78 g/kg respectively in week 6, and then declined only slightly further in the following 9 weeks. Adkins and Russel (*pers comm*) found no change in [BF] in the milk of feral goats during the first 10 weeks of lactation although the concentration of protein fell in parallel with that in the domestic goats.

In French breeds, the concentrations of both fat and protein were found to fall by about 10 g/kg as milk production increased from 300 to 1200 litres/lactation (Morand-Fehr *et al* 1986). In the same survey, fat concentration fell by 23 g/kg as parity rose from 1 to 8, but protein concentration was not affected.

2.2.2   Nitrogen fractions

The concentration of different nitrogen fractions in the milk of British breeds reported by Knowles and Watkin (1938) is shown in Table 2.12. The

Table 2.12: Concentration (g/kg) of certain nitrogen (N) fractions in goats' milk (Knowles and Watkin 1938).

Breed	Total N	Casein N	Albumin + globulin N	Non-protein N
Anglo-Nubian	6.03	4.56	0.86	0.61
Saanen	5.06	3.75	0.63	0.69
British Saanen	4.86	3.67	0.66	0.53
Toggenburg	4.86	3.54	0.74	0.56
British Toggenburg	5.34	4.00	0.58	0.77
British Alpine	5.13	3.75	0.60	0.78
British	4.95	3.61	0.52	0.83
English	5.45	3.98	0.91	0.55

distribution among the different fractions was fairly similar between breeds, and casein N varied from 0.73 to 0.76 of total N. In other reports covering European breeds, the proportion of casein N varied from about 0.70 to 0.79 (Parkash and Jenness 1968; Jenness 1980; Morand-Fehr *et al* 1986; Badamana *et al* 1990), which can be compared with values of 0.76 to 0.79 for cows' milk (Parkash and Jenness 1968; ARC 1980). Estimates of the proportion of non-protein N (NPN) vary. Values in the range 0.10 to 0.17 (reflecting concentrations of 0.55 to 0.83 g NPN/kg milk) reported for British breeds in 1938 (Table 2.12) appear to be high relative to more recent estimates (Parkash and Jenness 1968; Jenness, 1980; Morand-Fehr *et al* 1986; Badamana *et al* 1990; Sutton and Cook, *unpub*) where the majority of values are closer to 0.10, giving NPN concentrations in the range 0.30 to 0.50 g/kg milk. AFRC (1993) adopted 0.1 NPN in total N when calculating the true protein content of goats' milk. In cows' milk, NPN is about 0.05 of total N (ARC 1980).

2.2.3 Minerals

The concentration of the major minerals in goats' milk of European breeds under temperate conditions is given in Table 2.13. There is reasonable agreement among the various reports for most of the minerals. No results have been located for the mineral composition of the milk of Angora, cashmere or feral goats.

Several reviewers have commented that the mineral composition of goats' milk is similar to that of cows' milk (Haenlein 1980a,b; Jenness 1980; Morand-Fehr and Sauvant 1980; NRC 1981; Kessler 1981). In Table 2.14, values from Table 2.13 for the two principal breed groups of UK goats are compared with recommended values (ARC 1980) for dairy cows and sheep. According to this, the concentrations of most minerals except Na are greater

Table 2.13: Mineral composition (g/kg) of the milk of European breeds in temperate conditions.

Breed	Concentration (g/kg)							Reference
	Ash	Ca	P	Mg	K	Na	Cl	
Anglo-Nubian	8.7	1.57	1.38	–	–	–	1.40	Knowles and Watkin (1938)
Saanen	6.9	1.32	0.96	–	–	–	1.67	Knowles and Watkin (1938)
British Saanen	7.2	1.26	1.03	–	–	–	1.57	Knowles and Watkin (1938)
Toggenburg	8.3	1.37	1.24	–	–	–	1.58	Knowles and Watkin (1938)
British Toggenburg	8.0	1.45	1.26	–	–	–	1.50	Knowles and Watkin (1938)
British Alpine	8.3	1.38	1.18	–	–	–	1.54	Knowles and Watkin (1938)
British	7.6	1.32	1.14	–	–	–	1.57	Knowles and Watkin (1938)
English	7.2	1.41	1.2	–	–	–	1.56	Knowles and Watkin (1938)
Alpinen Wildziegen	–	1.23 to 1.41	0.88 to 0.93	0.10 to 0.13	1.50 to 1.80	0.30 to 0.37	–	Maraval and Vignon (1982)
Saanen-Welsh	–	–	–	–	1.8	0.44	0.53	Linzell (1967)
Saanen-Toggenburg	–	–	–	–	2.41	0.4	1.36	Konar et al (1971)
Various	–	1.37	1.12	0.17	1.7	–	–	Holmes et al (1946)
Not given	–	1.38	0.95	0.21	1.93	0.38	2.04	Bosworth and Van Slyke (1916)
Not given	–	1.25	0.9	0.12	2	0.4	1.30	Gueguen et al (1988)
Saanen	–	–	–	0.13 to 0.14	2.05 to 2.12	0.42 to 0.43	–	Kessler (1981)

Table 2.14: Suggested values for fat and mineral concentrations in milk (g/kg) for two main breed groups of UK goats compared with ARC (1980) recommended values for dairy cows and sheep.

	Goat		Cow		Sheep
	Anglo-Nubian	Saanen/Toggenburg	Guernsey	British Friesian	
Fat	46.5	37.4	45.0	36.8	70.0
Calcium	1.6	1.3	1.3	1.13	1.6
Phosphorus	1.4	0.9	1.02	0.9	1.3
Magnesium[1]	–	0.13	–	0.125	0.17
Potassium[1]	–	2.0	1.54	1.58	1.4
Sodium[1]	–	0.4	0.48	0.58	0.4
Chlorine	1.4	1.6	0.96	1.13	1.1

[1] Dash indicates that no values have been located in the literature.

in the milk of goats than cows at similar milk fat levels.

There is a well established relationship between the butterfat and the Ca contents of cows' milk (ARC 1980). Although the correlation between Ca and protein contents appears to be better, until relatively recently protein contents were not routinely determined and the relationship was difficult to quantify. NRC (1981) recommended that for goats both the Ca and protein dietary allowances should be increased as the butterfat content of the milk increased, although ARC (1980) considered that for cattle the correlation between the butterfat content of milk and the concentration of minerals other than Ca was too weak to be of predictive value. The recommended prediction equation in ARC (1980) for cows' milk is:

$$\text{Ca concentration (g/kg)} = 0.79 + 0.011 \, [\text{BF}] \, (\text{g/kg})$$

According to this equation, the Ca concentration in the milk of Anglo-Nubian and Saanen/ Toggenburg goats respectively would be 1.3 and 1.2 g/kg, rather lower than the values of 1.6 and 1.3 g/kg in Table 2.14.

The mineral composition of colostrum varies markedly from that of milk, and Maraval and Vignon (1982) found that concentrations of Ca (1.9 g/kg), P (1.5 g/kg) and Mg (0.24 g/kg) in the first milk produced by lactating goats was considerably higher than for milk produced later in lactation. Values fell to 1.3 g Ca, 0.9 g P and 0.12 g Mg/kg milk after 2 weeks and there was a further, slow fall up to 7 weeks (Table 2.13).

Other observations (Mba 1982) suggest that the Na and K contents of milk increase and decrease respectively with advancing lactation, and that Ca and P contents are also influenced by stage of lactation and are inversely related to milk yield.

2.2.4   Energy value

Many equations have been developed for predicting the energy value [EV$_1$] of milk from the concentration of its solids components, particularly butterfat. In ARC (1980) an equation developed by Tyrrell and Reid (1965) was proposed for cows' milk, with a quite different equation, from Brett *et al* (1972), for ewes' milk. The latter has a higher fat content than cow's milk but values are within the range for certain UK breeds of goat, including feral goats.

No prediction equation appears to have been developed for goats' milk from experimentally determined values for [EV$_1$]. Comparisons of different computational approaches to predicting the [EV$_1$] of goats' milk have been published (Economides 1986; Mavrogenis and Papachristoforou 1988), but only Morand-Fehr and Sauvant (1978b) have reported comparison of measured [EV$_1$] values with those from a prediction equation. From unpublished results they recommended the following equation, which is based on, and very similar to, one of Gaines' several equations (see Tyrrell and Reid 1965) for cows' milk:

$$[EV_1]\ (kJ/kg) = 1309 + 49.25[BF]$$

where [EV$_1$] = energy concentration (kJ/kg)
  and [BF] = butterfat concentration (g/kg).

Milk composition is increasingly being reported in the UK in terms of the concentrations of only butterfat [BF] and protein [P] as percent per litre, (g/kg milk = % per litre × 9.71). In view of the broad similarity of the composition of the milk of the dairy goat to that of the dairy cow, and the similarity of the prediction equations for the energy value of cows' and goats' milk according to Morand-Fehr and Sauvant (1978b), it is proposed that the following prediction equation from Tyrrell and Reid (1965) for cows' milk, should also be adopted for the [EV$_1$] of goats' milk:

$$[EV_1]\ MJ/kg = 0.0376[BF] + 0.0209[P] + 0.948$$

where [BF] is butterfat and [P] is milk protein concentration, both as g/kg milk.

This equation was developed from cows' milk with butterfat concentrations ranging from 16 to 64 g/kg. There is no evidence to indicate what error may be involved in applying these equations to the milk of goats such as feral goats, where the milk fat concentration may reach 70 g/kg (Russel and Adkins 1990). There is a clear need for direct measurements of the [EV$_1$] of goats' milk of widely varying composition, for the development of prediction equations specifically for goats or, alternatively, to validate the use of equations developed for cows' milk.

2.3 Fibre

2.3.1 Types of fibre

Goat fibres grow from the primary and secondary skin follicles. The primary follicles are the larger of the two types and typically occur in groups of three in association with a greater number of the smaller secondary follicles. The ratio of the number of secondaries to primaries (the S/P ratio) can vary between goats from less than 4 : 1 to more than 9 : 1, animals with the higher ratio generally having higher levels of production.

Most goats produce two types of fibre – a coarse outer coat of "guard hair" from the primary follicles and a fine "undercoat" or "down" from the secondary follicles. The guard hair has a mean fibre diameter of around 80 μm and is of little or no commercial value. Whether or not the fine undercoat can be classified as cashmere depends on the buyer as there is no internationally agreed definition of this product. In the UK, goat hair from secondary follicles which has an approximately normal distribution of fibre diameter with a mean value of less than about 19 μm and no fibres of more than 28 μm would generally be regarded as cashmere. In other countries the definition is less precise. The undercoat from dairy goats probably conforms to the strictest definition of cashmere, but the quantity produced per animal is negligible and the length of the fibre is too short for it to have any commercial value. In cashmere goats both types of fibre grow seasonally and are shed annually.

Mohair is produced only by Angora goats. (The fibre termed *angora* is produced by a breed of rabbit, and is outside the remit of this report.) This breed of goat is probably unique in growing fibres of approximately the same diameter from both primary and secondary follicles, although some primaries may produce coarser medullated fibres which are regarded as a fault and which downgrade the value of the fleece. The Angora can thus be regarded as a single-coated goat. Unlike cashmere goats, the Angora grows fibre continuously throughout the year. Mohair is coarser than cashmere, ranging in mean fibre diameter from 23 μm or less in super-fine kid mohair to 40 μm or more in strong adult hair.

For the sake of completeness, mention must be made of a third type of goat fibre which has appeared as a new product on the world market in recent years. This is known as *cashgora* and, as the name implies, comes from the cross-bred progeny of cashmere (or dairy goat) and Angora matings. The mean fibre diameter is generally 19 to 23 μm, but the distribution of fibre diameter is not normal, there being a secondary peak towards the upper end of the range. In the UK, *cashgora* comes from the early generations of "grading-up" dairy goats to "pure" Angoras by repeated crossings with Angora bucks, but in some eastern countries it has probably been produced for many years as a result of the occasional use of Angoras to increase the fibre production of cashmere goats. Cashgora goats, like those producing cashmere, have a double coat, with both types of fibre growing seasonally and being shed annually. Cashgora production is not considered specifically in this report.

2.3.2 Composition of and nutrient retention in goat fibre

All goat hair, like other animal fibres, is a complex mixture of proteins of the α-keratin family. These proteins are rich in the sulphur (S)-containing amino acid cystine which, in non-ruminants, is an essential dietary constituent for normal hair growth. In goats, as in other ruminants, cystine is synthesised by the rumen micro-organisms from methionine.

In addition to the one or more types of hair described above, the goat fleece also contains waxes secreted from the sebaceous glands and suint from the sweat glands associated with the primary follicles. The suggested chemical constituents of these products are given in Table 2.15, based on data for the chemical composition of sheep fleeces given by ARC (1980).

The wax or grease content of goat fleeces is substantially less than the figure of 12% generally applied to the wool of British sheep breeds (ARC 1980); the grease content of cashmere is typically of the order of 2 to 3%, while that of mohair varies from about 4 to 8% depending on the strain of Angora from which it comes (Smith *pers comm*).

Values for the production of suint, which has a particularly high concentration of K salts, are more difficult to obtain as the constituents of suint are soluble and more likely to be washed out of goat fleeces than wool by rain. In the absence of reliable data, a figure of 8% of the clean fibre yield has been used, although it is probable that suint production is related more closely to body weight than to fleece weight. The contents of the principal nutrients in the secretions associated with fibre production are small in relation to those of the fibre itself and are negligible in respect of the whole

Table 2.15: Proportions of the components of goat hair and associated secretions and the chemical composition of wool components as stated by ARC (1980).

| Component | Relative proportions | Chemical constituent (g/kg) | | | | | | | Energy (MJ/kg DM) |
		N	S	Ca	P	Mg	K	Na	
Fibre	0.84–0.90	165	33	1	0.1	0.1	0.05	0.3	23.5
Wax: Cashmere	0.02–0.03[1]	1.5	–	0.3	0.8	0.1	6.8	0.3	40.8
Angora	0.04–0.08[1]								
Suint	0.08[2]	27	4	7	1.2	2	200	10	–

[1] G.A. Smith *pers comm.*
[2] ARC (1980).

Table 2.16: Nutrient retention in hair and associated secretions during goat fibre production.

Breed	Scoured fibre weight		Nutrient retention (mg/d)							Energy retention, $(E_{w,}$ kJ/d)
	kg/year	g/d	N	S	Ca	P	Mg	K	Na	
Cashmere	0.625[1]	3.4[2]	573[2]	114[2]	5[2]	1[2]	1[2]	56[2]	4[2]	84[2]
Angora	3.5	9.6	1604	320	15	2	3	158	11	249

[1] 250 g down, 40% yield.
[2] June to December in cashmere goats.

animal's requirements for, and retention of nutrients.

The figures on nutrient retention in goat fibre and its associated secretions given in Table 2.16 have been calculated from data presented by ARC (1980) for wool. It should be noted that the calculations made using the above assumptions give a value for N retention in the fibre production of dairy goats which, during the period of fibre growth, is approximately 50% that of the figure presented in Section 6.9.3, for dermal N losses, or 25% of those losses calculated on an annual basis. The difference may be due, at least in part, to N losses in scurf. The nutrient retention figures for dairy and cashmere goats assume that fibre growth occurs from June to December and that mohair grows at a constant rate throughout the year. Neither assumption is wholly valid, but the consequent errors are considered to be negligible.

3.   Digestive Physiology

Digestive processes are central to the control of feed intake and meeting the animal's nutrient requirements. This short section is included in view of the frequent suggestions in the literature that in goats, digestive processes may differ in important aspects from those of cattle and sheep.

3.1   Digestibility

A large number of comparisons have been undertaken between sheep and goats (see reviews by Devendra 1978; Ndosa 1980; McCammon-Feldman *et al* 1981; Wahed 1984; Tan 1988). Many of the experiments have been undertaken in the tropics and can be criticised for reasons similar to those given in Section 4 for intake studies. Evidence is generally inconclusive and does not support the popular belief that feeds are better digested by goats than by sheep.

Well-replicated experiments at Reading University involving a range of feeds and levels of feeding (Ndosa (1980) with pelleted dried grass, and medium- and low-digestibility grass hay; Mohammed (1982) with pelleted dried lucerne) have shown no differences between the apparent digestibilities of organic matter (OM) in sheep and goats. The study of Alam *et al* (1983) showed that values for sheep may decline over time (after about 10 weeks), relative to those for goats, when given low-quality roughages without supplementation. Subsequent work by Alam *et al* (1987) also showed no differences in the partitioning of digestion of DM, neutral detergent fibre (NDF) or non-ammonia N in the digestive tract between kids and lambs given high-quality meadow hay. On the other hand, the recent study by Domingue *et al* (1991) showed that unsupplemented prairie grass straw (13.7 g N/kg DM) was better digested by goats than by sheep.

3.2   Rumen ammonia and rate of digestion

Several studies (Watson and Norton 1982; Cabrera *et al* 1983, Hadjipanayiotou and Antoniou 1983; Antoniou and Hadjipanayiotou 1985; Domingue *et al*
1991) have shown goats to have higher rumen ammonia concentrations than
sheep when fed on low-quality roughages. Alam *et al* (1985) concluded that
this was why goats had a higher digestible OM intake when offered forages
with OM digestibilities of less than 60%.

Tan *et al* (1987), however, showed that the higher intake of digestible OM
and higher rumen ammonia concentration in goats were not associated with
a higher rate of digestion in the rumen when feeding unsupplemented barley
straw was given to sheep and goats. In fact, 24- and 48-hour DM degradation
of straw suspended in the rumen of goats was lower than with sheep. Rate of
digestion studies with sheep and goats fed on high-quality forages do not
seem to have been undertaken. Nevertheless, various studies (Pant *et al* 1962;
Gihad 1979; Cabrera *et al* 1983; Alrahmoun *et al* 1985) have indicated that
goat rumen fluid may be more cellulolytic and have a greater microbial
population size than that of sheep. However, rumen fluid samples are unlikely
to be representative of total rumen contents.

3.3   Rate of passage and rumen volume

Huston (1978) and McCammon-Feldman *et al* (1981) cited Castle (1956) in
suggesting that the rate of passage of stained feed particles was more rapid
in goats than in sheep and cattle. However, Castle's study only involved goats.
Direct comparison of sheep and goats by Ndosa (1980) and Doyle and Egan
(1980) indicated a slower rate of passage in goats. Masson *et al* (1986) also
showed the rate to be marginally lower in goats. The results of Ndosa (1980)
and Doyle and Egan (1980) are contrary to expectation in view of the fact that
they observed a higher daily feed DM intake by goats than in sheep.

Rumen fill is known to increase with level of intake (e.g. Bines *et al* 1969;
Weston and Cantle 1982), thus differences in fill observed between species
need cautious interpretation. Nevertheless, studies by Watson and Norton
(1982) who used immature or mature pangola grass, by Gamble and
Mackintosh (1982) who used a mixture of lucerne hay and oat chaff, by Tan
(1988) who used barley straw, and by Domingue *et al* (1991) who used low-
quality prairie grass straw showed rumen fluid volume in relation to live
weight to be higher in goats than in sheep. This could explain why goats seem
able to consume more digestible OM than sheep, without having higher rates
of passage or faster rates of digestion.

3.4   Conclusions

From the evidence reviewed, it appears that goats and sheep have similar capacities to digest forages of medium to high digestibility (OM digestibility >60%). When fed on low-quality roughages without supplementation with N, goats are likely to be at an advantage over sheep in being able to maintain digestibility, possible due to a higher concentration of rumen ammonia. Rate of passage appears to be slower and rumen volume larger in goats compared to sheep.

An important consequence is that conventional feeds (i.e. excluding low-quality roughages fed without N supplements) are likely to have the same digestible energy value, [DE] and presumably metabolisable energy value [ME] value, for both sheep and goats.

4. Feed Intake

4.1 Introduction

Given the lack of British goat data and the voluminous literature on cattle and sheep (ARC 1980), a primary objective of the Working Party was to assess whether sheep (and possibly cattle) standards for intake are applicable to goats. Thus species comparisons for intake were reviewed. The question of whether goats have any unique feeding habits relative to sheep and cattle was also considered because of its implications for inter-species extrapolation. A further objective was to examine whether any goat intake standards are available elsewhere, and if so whether they are likely to be useful under UK conditions.

4.2 Feeding behaviour

Simpson (1945) and Gentry (1978) (cited by Van Soest 1982) classified goats as "intermediate browsers", sheep as "grazers" and cattle as "bulk and roughage eaters". Lu (1988) has recently described goats as "mixed-feeding opportunists" (see Section 4.3). Both goats and sheep are considered more capable of selective feeding than cattle because of their cleft upper lips (Hafez 1975). Goats, however, are notoriously selective and adaptive feeders, as judged by grazing/browsing studies (French 1970; McCammon-Feldman *et al* 1981; Merrill and Taylor 1981; Lu and Coleman 1986). Compared to sheep and cattle, goats have a greater tolerance to bitterness (Goatcher and Church 1970), thus they will consume shrub and tree leaves which are normally rejected by the other two species. A grazing comparison of sheep and goats in Scotland (Grant *et al* 1984) showed sheep to graze similar proportions of grass and clover leaves whereas goats grazed a lower proportion of clover leaves (see also Section 4.3).

Even under stall-feeding conditions goats and sheep are capable of selective feeding, as shown by Wahed and Owen (1986a). In this study the experiments involved feeding lucerne hay or ammonia-treated barley straw *ad libitum* and allowing the animals to refuse 20% of the amount offered.

Under this regime there was no clear evidence that goats were more selective than sheep, but goats had higher intakes than sheep. Further studies (Wahed and Owen 1986b; Wahed 1987) with goats fed untreated barley straw showed intakes to increase by a third when animals were allowed to refuse 50% of the amount offered instead of 20%. The intake response was judged to be due to goats being able to select more leaf and less stem with the higher rate of straw offered.

Another study at Reading (Naate 1986) showed a similar response with sheep, but apart from Wahed and Owen (1986a) a direct comparison of goats and sheep has not been made. The INRA standards (Morand-Fehr and Sauvant 1988) also drew attention to the ability of the goat to feed selectively and the consequent implications for deriving feed intake standards, particularly for forage feeds.

4.3   Grazing

The goat's grazing behaviour and diet selection are markedly different from those of other species of farmed livestock. Lu (1988), in a review of this subject, considered the classification of goats as browsers or grazers to be equivocal and suggested that they should be termed "mixed-feeding opportunists". They harvest material from a wide range of plant species and, at the same, time exhibit marked preferences as regards the parts of any particular species which they select. Given the opportunity they will browse trees and shrubs to a considerably greater extent than will sheep or cattle (McMahon 1964; Bell 1973), and their preferential selection of what are commonly regarded as weed species in modern agricultural systems has led to their use in the manipulation and improvement of both indigenous and sown pasture (e.g. Rolston *et al* 1981; Clark *et al* 1982; Radcliffe 1982; Russel *et al* 1983; Grant *et al* 1984). It is well established that goats can survive and indeed flourish in areas where cattle and sheep cannot (Lu 1988). However, with goats grazing sown swards under either rotational or set-stocked regimes, levels of herbage intake and performance appear to be more sensitive to herbage mass and sward height than is the case with sheep (McCall and Lambert 1987). As herbage mass declines the DM intake of goats (estimated from the rate of disappearance of herbage mass) declines at a faster rate than that observed in sheep or cattle, and goats appear virtually to stop grazing at a herbage mass of about 1000 kg DM/ha (Collins and Nicol 1986). Information on the effects of pasture allowance or sward height on DM intake and milk production in dairy goats is sparse. Evidence from the work of Jagusch and Kidd (1982) (cited by McCall and Lambert 1987), albeit with Saanens producing 1 to 3 litres milk/d, indicated that increases in apparent intake and milk production are obtained with pasture allowances up to 8 to 9 kg DM/head per day in early lactation and up to 6 to 7 kg DM/head per day in late lactation. Herbage intakes were estimated to be 3.0 to 3.3 and 1.8 to 2.0 kg DM/head per day respectively. Responses were greater in early rather than late lactation.

McCall and Lambert (1987) reported work on the effect of pasture allowance on the performance of pregnant and lactating cashmere goats. They concluded that an allowance of 1.5 kg DM/doe per day, or a pasture residual DM of 1300 kg DM/ha (sward height of 4 cm) appeared to be satisfactory for grazing does in late pregnancy. During lactation the live-weight gains of does and kids increased as herbage mass increased from 1250 to 2600 kg DM/ha and sward height from 2 to 7 cm. Even higher sward heights may give further increases in production; Nicol and Russel (*pers comm*) noted a significant response in the live-weight gains of yearling cashmere goats to an increase in sward height from 8 to 12 cm.

4.4   Species comparisons: stall-feeding, minimum selection

The difficulty of inter-species extrapolation is illustrated by data reviewed by ARC (1980). Mean intakes relative to body weight (W) of DM (g DM/kgW$^{0.75}$ daily) of coarse diets (roughages excluding grass silages) by growing sheep (54.9 g) are considerably lower than those by growing cattle (82.7 g), the difference between species being greater the smaller the sheep and the lower the forage digestibility. With grass silages the differences are larger because of low silage DM intakes by sheep.

There appear to be no direct feed intake comparisons of goats and cattle, but there are many involving goats and sheep, as reviewed by Wahed (1987) and Tan (1988). With the exception of studies in France (Simiane *et al* 1981) and New Zealand (Alam *et al* 1983, 1985; Tan 1988; Howe *et al* 1988), most have been carried out in the tropics with tropical breeds and feeds. None involved lactating animals and hardly any involved growing animals. The experiments were generally poorly designed, involving too few replicates and poorly-matched species representatives (e.g. differing in age, weight or potential mature size).

Simiane *et al* (1981) undertook a total of 41 intake and digestibility comparisons of mutton sheep (presumably adult castrates) and non-lactating goats fed on green forages, silages and hays of varying quality. Overall mean intakes were 55.8 and 65.3 g DM/kgW$^{0.75}$ daily for sheep and goats respectively. Goat intakes were 17% higher than those of sheep.

Intake studies at Reading University (Table 4.1) showed larger differences between sheep and goats. The well-replicated studies (in different experiments) involved castrate adult sheep and goats of comparable ages (9 to 24 months) and weight. Overall, mean intakes were 59.6 and 76.8 g

Table 4.1: Intake comparisons of goats and sheep in experiments with adult castrates at Reading University.

Reference	Feed type	Organic matter digestibility [OMD] (g/kg)[1]	Daily dry matter intake (g/kg $W^{0.75}$)	
			Goats[2] mean (n)	Sheep[3] mean (n)
Ndosa (1980)	Pelleted dried grass	690	121.4 (8)	99.1 (8) 89.4 (4)
	Grass hay	550	78.0 (8)	59.1 (8) 60.0 (4)
	Grass hay	510	73.9 (8)	53.6 (8) 53.2 (4)
	Barley straw and soyabean meal[4]	300[5]	65.3 (8)	47.5 (8) 41.4 (4)
Ndosa (1980)	Grass hay	550	74.6 (5)	50.6 (5)
Wahed (1984)	Barley straw and concentrate[6]	440[5]	59.0 (8)	53.0 (12)
Wahed (1984)	Lucerne hay	640	84.7 (10)	75.9 (10)
Wahed (1984)	Ammoniated barley straw	630	57.7 (8)	45.3 (8)

[1] *In vitro.*
[2] Saanen.
[3] For Ndosa (1980) n=8 were Welsh Mountain and n=4 were Suffolk × Scotch Halfbred. In all other trials the sheep were Suffolk × Mule.
[4] Straw 71.5% and soyabean meal 28.5% of the diet.
[5] Straw digestibility.
[6] Straw 90% and concentrate 10% of the diet.

DM/kg$W^{0.75}$ daily for sheep and goats respectively, goat intakes being 29% higher than those for sheep. In these studies and in those of Simiane *et al* (1981), the higher intake of goats is considered to be a reflection of their higher maintenance energy requirements, as shown by other studies at Reading (Mohammed and Owen 1981,1982) and at Edinburgh (Roy-Smith 1980). Tan (1988), in New Zealand, also came to this conclusion to explain the higher intakes of goats.

The dearth of direct comparisons of growing kids and lambs has been noted earlier. The one study at Reading University by Mohammed (1982) (Table 4.2) showed post early-weaning growth rates of kids to be only half those of lambs reared similarly. In this trial even the growth rate of the lambs was lower than expected, which may have reflected the apparent reluctance of the lambs to consume the lucerne pellets, especially at weaning. Daily intakes of the kids were somewhat lower than those of the lambs, presumably reflecting a lower growth potential of the kids used, and again illustrating the difficulty of making inter-species comparisons.

Alam *et al* (1983) in New Zealand compared the intake and digestibility

Table 4.2: Intake and growth comparisons at Reading University for artificially-reared kids and lambs individually fed *ad libitum* on dried lucerne pellets (Mohammed 1982).

	Castrated Saanen kids	Suffolk × (Cadzow Improver × Scottish Blackface) lambs
Number of animals	8	8
Age (days) at 10 kg live weight[1]	42	29
Growth rate (g/d) from 10 kg to approximately 23 kg live weight	106	205
Lucerne[2] dry matter intake (g/d)	752	825

[1] After weaning.
[2] 168 g crude protein/kg DM, 590 g/kg [OMD] *in vitro.*

of hay by feral × Saanen kids (mean weight 13.3 kg) and Dorset Down lambs (mean weight 20.5 kg), both approximately four months of age initially. Intakes of milled meadow hay over 12 weeks were similar for the two species (50.0 and 50.1 g $DM/kgW^{0.75}$ daily for the kids and lambs, respectively) and both maintained their weights over the period. Apparent DM digestibilities of the hay were similar for the two species during the fourth and sixth weeks of the experiment, but in the tenth week DM digestibility by the kids was superior (60 *vs* 55%) and was considered to be a reflection of the superior ability of goats to maintain their digestive capacity when fed low-N feed (the hay contained 7.1 g N/kg DM). During weeks 13 to 16, when milled lucerne was fed, the intake of the lambs tended to be higher than that of the kids (84 *vs* 73 g $DM/kgW^{0.75}$ daily) and feed dry matter digestibilities were comparable (60 *vs* 59%). In subsequent experiments (Alam *et al* 1985) with the same animals fed a range of forages, digestible organic matter (OM) intakes were higher for goats when forage OM digestibility was less than 60%. Similar findings in New Zealand were recently reported by Domingue *et al* (1991) who used prairie grass straw (13.7 g N/kg DM). Dry matter intakes (56 *vs* 36 g/kgW$^{0.75}$ daily) and DM digestibilities (36.8 *vs* 32.6%) were higher for goats than sheep.

It is concluded that voluntary feed intakes by adult goats are usually greater than those by sheep, but the size of the difference is variable. There is insufficient evidence to draw any conclusions about the relative intakes of kids and lambs.

4.5 Published estimates of feed intake by goats

The published estimates of the voluntary feed intake of goats include NRC (1981) for the USA, Kearl (1982) for developing countries, Skjevdal (1982) for Norway and the French standards (Morand-Fehr 1981; Morand-Fehr *et al*

1987; Morand-Fehr and Sauvant 1988). The NRC (1981) nutrient standards, which are specifically for goats, do not consider intake *per se*, nor did the article by Skjevdal (1982) which discussed Norwegian nutrient standards.

Kearl (1982) considered the nutrient requirements of ruminants in developing countries and included separate sections on goats and sheep. Literature from both developed regions (mainly France) and developing ones (especially India) were reviewed and a "mean" DM intake value for each species and physiological state was calculated. For goats, values were 76.7, 76.3 and 119.6 g DM/kgW$^{0.75}$ daily for growth, late pregnancy and lactation respectively. For comparison, values for sheep were, respectively, 74.9, 90.0 and 138.0 g DM/kgW$^{0.75}$ daily. For growing goats and sheep, intake variations due to differences in dietary metabolisable energy concentrations [ME] as Mcal/kg DM were adjusted by an "*F*" factor where:

$$F = -0.666 + 1.333[ME] - 0.2666[ME]^2$$

where [ME] is as Mcal/kg DM.

Thus for growing goats fed a diet with an energy concentration of 1.78 Mcal (7.44 MJ) ME/kg DM the "*F*" factor would be 0.86 and feed intake would be 66.0 g DM/kgW$^{0.75}$ daily. Except for growth, it is interesting that the "averages" derived show intakes to be generally higher for goats than for sheep. Species comparisons derived in this way are relatively meaningless, however, as they reflect many other differences, notably in performance potential and diet.

It is clear that the only substantial body of data available on the intake of lactating goats relevant to UK conditions are from France (Morand-Fehr 1981; Morand-Fehr and Sauvant 1988), which concentrate on adult dairy goats. Morand-Fehr (1981) claimed that in mid-lactation (weeks 10 to 30) the DM intake of grass or lucerne hay based diets was well predicted by the following equation (as modified by Alderman 1982):

$$DMI \ (kg/d) = 0.42Y + 0.024W^{0.75} + 0.4\Delta W + 0.7F_p$$

where Y   = milk yield in kg/d at 3.5% milk fat, W = live weight in kg,
    ΔW = live-weight change in kg/month
and F_p = proportion of forage as a decimal.

The equation was used to predict the intakes observed in four experiments undertaken in Reading and involving a total of 103 individually fed lactating goats (Table 4.3). The experiment of Sutton and Mowlem (1989) involved 29 goats, while the other experiments involved 7 to 9 goats per treatment.

Overall, the observed intakes were 14% higher than those predicted using the equation modified by Alderman (1982) (prediction A, Table 4.3) but there was a high correlation (r = 0.81) between the observed and predicted values.

Table 4.3: Observed dry matter (DM) intakes of lactating goats in experiments at the Institute of Grassland and Environmental Research, Shinfield, compared with intakes predicted using the equation of Morand-Fehr (1981) (as modified by Alderman 1982) and INRA (1988), Table 11.3.

Liveweight, W (kg)	Liveweight change, ΔW (kg/30 d)	Lactation week no. (n)	Milk yield (kg/d)	Forage Type	Forage F	Total DM intake (kg/d)	Predicted DM intake (kg/d) A	B	C
65.1	-0.09	3 to 11	2.82	Lucerne hay[1]	0.65	2.36	2.16	2.19	2.28
67.5	-0.64	3 to 11	2.96	Lucerne hay[2]	0.64	2.31	2.00	2.26	2.36
71.1	0.11	26 to 28	1.20	Barley straw[3]	0.55	1.54	1.52	1.47	1.88
64.2	0.12	26 to 28	1.61	Treated straw[3]	0.62	1.86	1.70	1.66	1.90
67.9	0.09	26 to 28	1.98	Grass hay[3]	0.65	2.00	1.89	1.85	2.07
62.9	-0.17	3 to 12	2.44	Grass hay[4]	0.55	1.99	1.88	1.95	2.13
60.4	-1.67	3 to 12	2.93	Grass silage[4]	0.49	1.76	1.42	2.09	2.24
65.1	-1.15	3 to 12	2.94	Hay/silage[4]	0.52	1.91	1.69	2.15	2.32
65.4	-1.26	4 to 15	2.54	Grass hay[5]	0.58	2.08	1.52	2.02	2.20
66.5	-0.63	4 to 15	2.67	Grass hay[6]	0.57	2.07	1.83	2.08	2.26
68.3	-0.42	4 to 15	2.58	Grass hay[7]	0.61	2.25	1.91	2.08	2.26
Means					0.58	2.01	1.77	1.98	2.17

F: Proportion of forage in total DM consumed.
A: Using the equation of Morand-Fehr (1981) as modified by Alderman (1982).
B: As A, but omitting the adjustment for live-weight change (ΔW).
C: Interpolated from Table 11.3 of INRA (1988), 2nd month of lactation to drying off.

References and diet details:

[1] Sutton and Mowlem (1989) Barley and soyabean meal concentrate.
[2] Sutton and Mowlem (1989) Molassed sugar beet pulp and soyabean meal concentrate.
[3] Sibanda et al (1989) Same concentrate fed with hay, straw and treated straw.
[4] Badamana (1987) Same concentrate fed with hay, silage and hay/silage mixture.
[5] Badamana (1987) Concentrate contained 117 g crude protein/kg DM.
[6] Badamana (1987) Concentrate contained 152 g crude protein/kg DM.
[7] Badamana (1987) Concentrate contained 185 g crude protein/kg DM.

The closest agreement between observed and predicted values occurred for the data of Sibanda *et al* (1989) with goats in mid to late lactation, which is the type of animal for which the equation was derived. The other experiments in Table 4.3 involved goats in early lactation, with the animals exhibiting a loss of weight. It is interesting that for these experiments, averaged over the 11 treatments, there was close agreement between the observed intakes and those predicted (prediction B, Table 4.3) if the live-weight change factor, ΔW, was omitted from the equation. The equation appears useful, but it needs corroborating with further data from the UK before conclusions on its applicability can be made.

The later French feed intake standards for goats (Morand-Fehr and Sauvant 1988) concentrate on adult dairy goats. They gave estimates of pregnant and lactating goat DM intakes, derived from INRA fill unit (UEL) values (Tables 4.4 and 4.5). In a preview published in 1987 (Morand-Fehr *et al* 1987) it was explained that the standards were based on an update of earlier data (Morand-Fehr and Sauvant 1978a) and they incorporate the INRA "fill unit" (unites d'encombrement; UE) system for predicting the voluntary intake

Table 4.4: Dry matter intakes of dry and pregnant goats using the French UEL System (Morand-Fehr and Sauvant 1988), based on diets of maize silage, lucerne hay and concentrate supplements.

Live-weight (kg)	Month of gestation	UEL[1]	Dry matter intake (kg/d)
40	Dry	1.52	1.07
	1 to 3	1.52	1.07
	4	1.52	1.07
	5	1.43	0.97
50	Dry	1.62	1.20
	1 to 3	1.62	1.20
	4	1.62	1.20
	5	1.53	1.09
60	Dry	1.72	1.33
	1 to 3	1.72	1.33
	4	1.72	1.33
	5	1.61	1.21
70	Dry	1.82	1.47
	1 to 3	1.82	1.47
	4	1.82	1.47
	5	1.71	1.34
80	Dry	1.92	1.60
	1 to 3	1.92	1.60
	4	1.92	1.60
	5	1.79	1.46

[1] Unités d'encombrement lait (fill unit for milk = 123 g DM average pasture/kg $W^{0.75}$).

Table 4.5: Dry matter intakes of dairy goats during the second month of lactation and onwards using the French UEL system (Morand-Fehr and Sauvant 1988), based on diets of maize silage, lucerne hay and concentrate supplements.

Live-weight (kg)	Milk yield[1] (kg/d)	UEL[2]	Dry matter intake (kg/d)
50	1	1.86	1.50
	2	2.09	1.81
	3	2.32	2.11
	4	2.55	2.42
	5	2.78	2.72
	6	3.02	3.03
60	1	1.96	1.64
	2	2.19	1.94
	3	2.42	2.25
	4	2.65	2.55
	5	2.88	2.86
	6	3.11	3.16
70	1	2.06	1.77
	2	2.29	2.07
	3	2.52	2.38
	4	2.75	2.68
	5	2.99	2.99
	6	3.23	3.30

[1] Containing 35 g/kg butterfat, [BF].
[2] Unités d'Encombrement Lait (Fill Unit for Milk = 123 g DM average pasture/kg $W^{0.75}$).

of forage-based diets for ruminants (Jarrige *et al* 1986). The UE system data bank is largely based on intake studies using "standard" sheep and relating the intakes of different forages fed *ad libitum* to that achieved with a reference grass by assigning them "fill values". Thus 1.0 kg DM of the reference grass is defined as being one "fill unit" in a "standard" sheep. The intake capacity of "standard" cows (weighing 600 kg and yielding 25 kg/d of milk with a [BF] of 40 g/kg) was measured using the sheep reference grass and experiments were conducted to relate "sheep fill values" of forages to "cow fill values". This enabled use to be made of the data bank already collected for sheep. Other experiments defined the changes in the intake capacity of cows as affected by weight, age and production level and these measurements were subsequently used to derive the prediction equations now employed in the application of the system. It appears that there are only limited data on "goat fill values" of different forages, but the few experiments undertaken to compare sheep fill values and goat fill values suggested a similar relation to that between sheep fill values and cow fill values.

The decision was therefore taken by the Working Party to use the "milk fill unit" (Unites d'Encombrement Lait; UEL) for dairy goats. The ingestive capacity of a 60-kg goat at maintenance is given as 1.72 UEL, with an

adjustment of 0.1 UEL for each 10.0-kg difference in live weight. Maintenance intake capacity is also assumed during the first four months of
gestation, with 90% of maintenance capacity in the fifth month (Table 4.4).
From the second month of lactation, a 60-kg goat yielding 4.0 kg/d of milk
with a [BF] of 35 g/kg (a "standard" goat) is deemed to have an ingestive
capacity of 2.65 UEL, with an adjustment of 0.23 UEL for each 1.0 kg
difference in 3.5% milk fat yield. During weeks 1 to 4 respectively of
lactation, ingestive capacities are given as 0.72, 0.83, 0.90 and 0.95 that of the
second month of lactation. DM intake is calculated using the UEL values of
different ingredients to be fed in the given dietary situation. Tables 4.4 and 4.5
(in part from Morand-Fehr and Sauvant 1988) illustrate the intake capacity of
goats fed typical French diets, based on maize silage and lucerne hay with
some concentrate supplementation. Their feed DM intake data can be
accurately fitted by the following equation:

$$\text{DMI (kg/d)} = 0.062W^{0.75} + 0.305Y$$

where Y = milk yield in kg/d at 3.5% milk fat, W = live weight in kg.

DM intake values given in Tables 4.4 and 4.5 would therefore be different for
dietary ingredients other than maize silage and lucerne hay. The UEL system
also assigns fill values to concentrates, depending on the forages with which
they are fed and the energy status of the animal, i.e. they depend on
substitution rates, and indeed prediction of substitution rates appears to be the
major novelty of the revised (1988) UEL system.

It seems, therefore, that there is little that is specific to goats in the revised
UEL system. Indeed Morand-Fehr *et al* (1987) stressed that the UEL system
should be applied to goats with extreme caution; the reaction of cows and
goats to different forages might be different and it has not yet been possible
to test the system with goats on a range of diets. Application of the French
standards to UK dairy goats would also depend on assuming that UK forages
and UK goats have similar fill values and ingestive capacities, respectively,
to French ones. In the case of forages, there is considerable contrast in the
types used, with maize silage and lucerne hay being common in France, and
grass hay (with some grass silage) being fed in the UK. Predicted DM intake
values, derived from INRA Fill Unit (UEL) values, given in Table 11.3 of
INRA (1988), are on average 0.2 kg/d higher than DM intakes measured with
lactating dairy goats producing about 2 kg milk/d, offered a variety of mixed
diets at the Institute of Grassland and Environmental Research (estimate C in
Table 4.3).

4.6   Seasonal effects

It is increasingly acknowledged that seasonal variations in voluntary feed intake occur in sheep (Blaxter and Boyne 1982; Argo and Smith 1983; Forbes 1986). There is some evidence that this also occurs in goats (De Jong 1981; Ash 1986). The importance of this for different classes of goats under UK conditions is a matter for investigation.

4.7   Water intake

With non-lactating animals of comparable physiological state, there is consistent evidence (e.g. Ndosa 1980; Mohammed 1982; Wahed 1984; Alam *et al* 1983, 1985; Howe *et al* 1988; Tan 1988) to show that goats consume less water than sheep. Whilst this may have important implications in arid/semi-arid situations, it seems of little significance as far as goat feeding in the UK is concerned.

4.8   Conclusions and recommendations

4.8.1   *Dry matter intakes of growing (weaned) kids*

In the absence of convincing evidence to the contrary, it is proposed that ARC (1980) intake standards for growing lambs should be used for goat kids. This assumes that conventional feeds (containing adequate N for rumen microbial activity; see Section 6.2 *et seq*) are offered *ad libitum* with a refusal rate of not more than 15% of that offered.

There is a need for intake studies in the UK with growing kids of different breed and types fed diets used in commercial practice.

4.8.2   *Dry matter intakes of adults at maintenance*

INRA (1988) English text, p. 179, Table 11.1 gives values for the DM intake capacity of female goats (40 to 80 kgW) at maintenance, and in Table 11.6 for male goats for live weights (60 to 120 kgW). All the figures given for both sexes are accurately fitted by the following equation:

$$DMI (kg/d) = 0.522 + 0.0135W$$

It is proposed that this equation should be adopted for dairy-type stall-fed adult goats at maintenance. Under grazing conditions, particularly in winter, higher allowances are likely to be necessary and the extent of increase needs to be established by research.

There is no information on the intake of fibre-type goats in the UK and it is therefore tentatively proposed that ARC (1980) intake standards for sheep should be used for them.

4.8.3   Dry matter intakes of pregnant and lactating dairy goats

In the absence of any other temperate climate evidence with European milk breeds, it is proposed that the French UEL standards (Morand-Fehr and Sauvant 1988), converted to DMI as kg/d, should be used for pregnant and lactating dairy goats. The following equation (based on INRA 1988) may be used to predict voluntary DM intakes for lactating goats from the second month of lactation:

$$DMI \text{ (kg/d)} = 0.062W^{0.75} + 0.305Y$$

where Y = milk yield in kg/d at 3.5% milk fat, W = live weight in kg.

However, this equation is based on diets of maize silage, lucerne hay and concentrates and different factors may apply for other diets. Again, it is assumed that the forage feeding regime is "conventional" and *ad libitum*. Corroboration of the INRA (1988) standards under UK conditions and with more typical UK feeds needs to be undertaken.

4.8.4   Water intake

It is proposed that, in supplying water, similar guidelines as those given by ARC (1980) for the water intake of cattle and sheep should be followed for goats.

5.   Energy

In the UK the energy requirements for ruminants are expressed in terms of metabolisable energy (ME) in a system based on calorimetric studies made by Blaxter (1962) and set out in detail in ARC (1980). The system provides a set of rules which link tables of feed composition to calculations of the energy requirements of the animals. It is proposed to use the same system to define the energy requirements of goats in different physiological states and with different levels of performance. Where possible, values for calculating the requirements of goats have been derived from experimentation on goats. Frequently, however, because of the very limited amount of work on goats specific information is not available and it has been necessary to use values for cattle or sheep taken from ARC (1980).

5.1   Efficiencies of utilisation of metabolisable energy

As there is very little specific information for goats on the efficiencies of utilisation of ME (k) for various physiological processes, it is proposed that the preferred values for ruminants given by ARC (1980) and shown in Table 5.1 are used to calculate the ME requirements of goats at each stage of the productive cycle. The methods by which the efficiencies were derived and the reasons for adopting the particular values are set out in detail in ARC (1980).

5.2   Feeding level corrections for ME intake

The ME actually available to the animal, calculated as the sum of the ME (measured at maintenance) of the diet's component feeds, falls with increasing levels of feeding. ARC (1980) proposed two different mathematical models to correct for this effect, one for lactating dairy cows and one for growing and fattening cattle.

Table 5.1: Preferred values for the efficiency of utilisation of metabolisable energy of normal diets by ruminants (from ARC 1980).

Function	Efficiency when metabolisability (q_m) of diet is:			
	0.4	0.5	0.6	0.7
Maintenance (k_m)[1]	0.643	0.678	0.713	0.748
Pregnancy (k_c)	0.133 for all values of q_m			
Growth and fattening (k_f)				
(a) All diets[2]	0.318	0.396	0.474	0.552
(b) Pelleted diets[3]	0.475	0.477	0.479	–
Lactation (k_1)[4]	0.560	0.595	0.630	0.665

[1] $k_m = 0.35q_m + 0.503$ [3] $k_f = 0.024q_m + 0.465$
[2] $k_f = 0.78q_m + 0.006$ [4] $k_1 = 0.35q_m + 0.420$

5.2.1 Dairy cattle

For dairy cattle, the decline in the availability of ME to the animal is estimated by ARC (1980) to be 1.8% per unit increase in feeding level (L) above maintenance ME requirement, excluding any safety margin. The correction factor C_L for ME requirements is calculated as follows:

$$C_L = 1 + 0.018(L - 1)$$

where L is calculated as a multiple of maintenance ME requirement.

AFRC (1990) extended the use of this correction factor to lactating ewes, so for the sake of consistency, the ME requirements of lactating and pregnant goats in the tables of this report have been calculated using this correction factor also.

5.2.2 Growing and fattening cattle

For growing and fattening animals, ARC (1980) adopted the feeding level correction of Blaxter and Boyne (1970).The equation has the form:

$$R = B(1 - e^{-kl}) - 1$$

where R is the retention of net energy,
    and I is the intake of dietary ME,
    both scaled by the fasting metabolism of the animal (F).

The factors B and k are calculated from the various efficiencies of utilisation of ME of ARC (1980) as follows:

$$B = k_m/(k_m - k_f)$$
$$k = k_m \times \ln(k_m/k_f)$$

The ME requirements of growing goats given in the tables of this report have been calculated using these ARC (1980) functions.

5.3 Requirements for maintenance

The energy requirements for maintenance (M_m) can be derived in two ways: from calorimetric measurements of the heat production of fasted animals (F) divided by the efficiency of ME utilisation k_m, or from feeding trials in which animals are fed at several different levels of energy intake, enabling calculation of the intake of ME at zero weight change.

5.3.1 Efficiency of ME utilisation

ARC (1980) gives a function which relates the efficiencies of energy use for maintenance (k_m) to the ME concentration of the diet ME/GE or q_m (Table 5.1). For diets with metabolisabilities (q_m) of 0.4, 0.5, 0.6 and 0.7 this gives values for k_m of 0.643, 0.678, 0.714 and 0.750.

5.3.2 Requirements

Nine estimates of fasting metabolism (F) of adult goats have been published (Table 5.2). They show a considerable range in the estimates of fasting metabolism which, as Sauvant (1981) commented, cannot be explained by the information available in the papers on the types of animals, their physio-logical state or the particular techniques used to make the measurements. The mean of the nine estimates is 315 ± 21.4 kJ/kgW$^{0.75}$ daily. This is very similar to the value in ARC (1980) of 319 kJ/kgW$^{0.75}$ for the fasting metabolism of adult cattle derived from feeding trials, which for cattle weighing 500 to 600 kg corresponds closely with the preferred value of 0.53 MJ/kgW$^{0.67}$ daily derived from a regression of 88 estimations of fasting metabolism on live weight. Thus, the fasting metabolism of both cattle and goats appears to be substantially higher than that of sheep, for which ARC (1980) gave preferred values of 230 kJ/kgW$^{0.75}$ daily at 2 years of age and 215 kJ/kgW$^{0.75}$ daily at 4 years of age.

The fasting metabolism of 315 kJ/kgW$^{0.75}$ daily gives maintenance ME requirements (M_m) of 490, 465, 441 and 420 kJ ME/kgW$^{0.75}$ daily for dietary q_m values of 0.4, 0.5, 0.6 and 0.7.

Seventeen estimates of the maintenance ME requirements (M_m) of goats derived from feeding trials were found (Table 5.3). Although the variation between estimates is considerable, it is less than that for the estimates of

Table 5.2: Estimates of the fasting metabolism of goats.

Reference	Fasting metabolism (F) (kJ/kg $W^{0.75}$ daily)
Morgen *et al* (1906)	403
Orr and Magee (1923)	308
Ritzman *et al* (1936)	212
Brody (1945)	372
Mitchell (1962)	314
Armstrong and Blaxter (1965)	218
Fujihara *et al* (1973)	356
Roy-Smith (1980)	331
Prieto *et al* (1990)	324
Mean	315 ± 21.4

fasting metabolism. The mean value of 438 ± 10.9 kJ ME/kg$W^{0.75}$ daily is very close to the value of 441 kJ/kg$W^{0.75}$ daily for M_m estimated from the mean value of the estimates of fasting metabolism in Table 5.2 assuming that a diet with a metabolisability (q_m) of 0.6 ($k_m = 0.714$) is being eaten. These results of feeding trials therefore confirm that the fasting metabolism of adult goats is similar to that of cattle rather than that of sheep. If substantial differences are shown to exist in the body compositions of goats of different types and breeds (e.g. European dairy, tropical, Angora, cashmere) a systematic investigation of the maintenance requirements of goats would be desirable to assess if there are important differences in maintenance requirements between different types of goats.

There are two reports of estimates of the maintenance requirements of milk-fed kids. Jagusch *et al* (1983) estimated a value of 470 kJ/kg$W^{0.75}$ daily in Saanen kids fed on goats' milk and Sanz Sampelayo *et al* (1988) gave values for M_m of 444 and 427 kJ/kg$W^{0.75}$ daily for Granadina kids fed on goats' milk or a milk replacer. These values for young unweaned kids do not vary greatly from the values for weaned or adult goats (Table 5.3), but they differ considerably from the situation in sheep where ARC (1980) suggested a value for the fasting metabolism of unweaned lambs of 350 kJ/kg$W^{0.75}$ daily compared to 230 to 210 kJ/kg$W^{0.75}$ daily in adult sheep from 2 to over 4 years of age. Goats may be more analogous to cattle, for which ARC (1980) suggested much less difference between the fasting metabolism of 342 to 385 kJ/kg$W^{0.75}$ daily in calves on liquid diets and 319 kJ/kg$W^{0.75}$ daily in adult animals. More data are needed before recommendations can be made to modify maintenance ME requirements for milk- or milk replacer-fed kids.

Table 5.3: Estimates of the maintenance requirements of goats derived from feeding trials.

Reference	Maintenance requirement, (M_m), (kJ ME/kg $W^{0.75}$ daily)
Stohmann *et al* (1868)	460
Majumdar (1960b)	482
Devendra (1967)	378
Opstvedt (1967)	530
Flatt *et al* (1972)	418
Akinsoyinu (1974)	389
Winter and Gorsch (1974)	384
Skjevdal (1974)	489
Sauvant and Morand-Fehr (1977)	456
Itoh *et al* (1977)	365
Rajpoot (1978)	427
Singh and Sengar (1978)	460
Haenlein (1980a)	464
Sengar (1980)	474
Mohammed and Owen (1981)	434
Aguilera *et al* (1990)	401
Prieto *et al* (1990)	443
Mean	438 ± 10.9

5.4   Requirements for activity

5.4.1   *Efficiency of ME utilisation*

Activity is regarded as part of the maintenance requirement of ruminant animals in the ARC (1980) scheme, so that the same efficiency factor, k_m has been used to calculate the ME needed to cover the cost of muscular activity during standing and walking.

5.4.2   *Requirements*

Different authors have suggested very large increases in energy expenditure above maintenance (activity allowance, A) to cover the costs of walking during grazing and other activities. NRC (1981), without citing references or the basis of the calculations, suggested no increase above maintenance for housed goats, an increase of 25% under intensive grazing and tropical conditions, an increase of 50% on semi-arid rangeland and on slightly hilly land, and an increase of 75% on sparse grassland and on "mountainous transhumance pasture". Wilkinson and Stark (1987a) suggested, again without stating a reason, that requirements should be increased by 25% for goats grazing lowland pasture and by 50% for those on extensive hill and upland pastures. Morand-Fehr *et al* (1987), using information from Blaxter (1962) on the energy costs of activity in sheep and cattle, calculated that additional requirements for activity by goats are between 10 and 20% of maintenance on pasture, between 30 and 50% on rangeland and 50 to 80% in very dry zones.

ARC (1980) give an energy cost of activity (A) of 2.6 J/kg/m for horizontal movement in sheep, based on two mean values (2.5 and 2.9 J/kg/m). However, Taylor *et al* (1974), who worked with goats, give a value of 3.63 J/kg/m for the energy cost of running, whilst Lachica *et al* (1997), using a treadmill with varying slopes (-10% to $+10\%$), quote a mean energy cost for Granadina goats walking on the level of 3.35 J/kg/m. A preferred value of 3.5 J/kg/m is adopted here for the energy cost of walking on the level for goats.

ARC (1980) quote 28 J/kg/m as the energy cost for vertical movement in sheep, which agrees with the findings of Lachica *et al* (1997) of 31.7 J/kg/m. ARC (1980) also give an additional cost of standing of 10 kJ/kg daily, and the cost of one body position change (lying down and then standing up again) as 260 J/kg (Table 5.4). Calculations shown in Table 5.5 use mainly the values from ARC (1980), except the higher figure for the energy cost of walking of 3.5 J/kg/m adopted in this Report, and allows for 10 body position changes per day. Morand-Fehr *et al* (1987) suggested levels of activity that are typical of goats in different environments, ie: 3000 m/d walking on good pasture and 5000 m/d on good quality range. Prieto *et al* (1991) estimated that the mean distances walked by grazing goats were 6432 m/d in summer and 3482 m/d in autumn, depending on pasture availability. Values in Table 5.5 give similar estimates of the extra costs of activity to those of Morand-Fehr *et al* (1987), but are slightly lower than those suggested by NRC (1981) for good grazing conditions, and much higher than those suggested for mountainous regions.

Table 5.4: Estimates of the additional energy costs of activity (A) for 65-kg goats based on ARC (1980)[1] and Lachica *et al* (1997)[2].

Activity	Energy cost	Energy cost for 65-kg goat
Horizontal movement[2]	3.5 J/kg/m	0.238 MJ/km
Vertical movement[1]	28 J/kg/m	0.182 MJ/100 metre
Standing[1]	10 kJ/kg daily	0.650 MJ/d
One position change[1]	0.26 kJ/kg	0.017 MJ/change

5.5   Requirements for growth

5.5.1   Efficiency of ME utilisation

Although considerable differences exist in the energy cost of deposition of fat and protein, and there are great differences in the rates of deposition of these

Table 5.5: Energy costs calculated according to ARC (1980) and Lachica *et al* (1997) of goat activity (A), specified by Morand-Fehr *et al* (1987).

| Environment | Distance travelled (m) | | Energy cost (MJ/d) | Total energy cost[1] (MJ/d) | Proportion of fasting metabolism[2] |
	Horizontally	Vertically			
On pasture	3000		0.68		
		100[3]	0.18	1.36	0.19
Good quality range	5000		1.14		
		100[3]	0.18	1.82	0.25
Very arid range	20000		4.55		
		900	1.64	6.69	0.93
Mountainous range	20000		4.55		
		1500	2.73	7.78	1.08

[1] Including a cost of standing for 12 h/d of 0.325 MJ/d and allowing for 10 position changes per day, costing 0.17 MJ/d.
[2] Assuming a fasting metabolism of 315 kJ/kg $W^{0.75}$ daily (7.21 MJ/d) for a 65-kg goat.
[3] 100 m assumed, as Morand-Fehr *et al* (1987) gave no vertical distance ascended.

two tissues with age and weight, ARC (1980) reached the conclusion that little error would arise if the same values for efficiencies were used for changes in body composition in adult non-lactating ruminants and in young growing ones, provided that they were weaned and eating solid food. These values for the efficiency of utilisation of ME for growth and fattening (k_f) differ for pelleted and non-pelleted diets and are given in Table 5.1.

For ruminants on liquid diets of either milk or milk substitutes an efficiency for growth (k_f) of 0.70 was preferred by ARC (1980). Recent studies, however, have found widely differing efficiencies of conversion of feed ME to energy gain in liquid-fed goat kids. Jagusch *et al* (1983) found an efficiency on goats' milk of 0.45 while Sanz Sampelayo *et al* (1988) found an efficiency of 0.73 on goats' milk and of 0.58 on milk substitute, which they commented may not have had an optimal composition for rearing kids. Jagusch *et al* (1983) stated that their extremely low value could be due to a sub-clinical deficiency in the goats' milk or to the persistence of thermogenic brown fat. Work by Prieto *et al* (1993) suggests that these requirements for growth may be modified by the ambient temperature in which the kids are housed. The efficiencies of conversion of milk substitute by kids fed *ad libitum* from birth to 2 months of age were 0.52, 0.66 and 0.76 g of gain per g of milk substitute DM at ambient temperatures of 12, 20 and 30°C, respectively. These differing estimates of the efficiencies of use of ME for liquid-fed kids do not suggest that the value of 0.70 for liquid-fed ruminants of ARC (1980) should be altered to a specific value for kids.

5.5.2 Requirements

The composition and energy value [EV_g] of live-weight gain in growing kids and adult goats has been described in Sections 2.1 and 2.2 and Tables 2.2 to 2.6. Application of the ARC (1980) predicted efficiency of ME utilisation for growth and fattening (k_f) (Table 5.1) to these values, and using the energy retention model described in Section 5.2.2, gives estimates of the energy requirements for maintenance and growth in castrate male kids shown in Table 5.6.

Table 5.6: Energy requirements (MJ ME/d) for maintenance[1] and growth[2] in castrate male kids.

Body weight, W (kg)	Live-weight gain (kg/d)	Metabolisability (q_m) of diet		
		0.5	0.6	0.7
15	0	4.1	3.9	3.7
	0.1	6.3	5.8	5.3
	0.2	9.5	8.1	7.2
20	0	5.1	4.8	4.6
	0.1	7.6	7.0	6.5
	0.2	11.2	9.7	8.7
25	0	6.0	5.7	5.4
	0.1	8.9	8.2	7.6
	0.2	12.9	11.2	10.1
30	0	6.9	6.5	6.2
	0.1	10.2	9.3	8.7
	0.2	14.6	12.7	11.5

[1] Calculated from energy costs of fasting metabolism of 315 kJ/kg $W^{0.75}$ daily with the addition of 10% for activity, 5 kJ/kg daily for 12 h standing and 1.7 kJ/kg daily for 10 position changes.
[2] Calculated from data in Table 2.4 and energy retention model of ARC (1980) for cattle.

5.6 Requirements for pregnancy

5.6.1 Efficiency of ME utilisation

ARC (1980) suggested a value of 0.133 for the efficiency of utilisation of ME for the production and maintenance of the conceptus (k_c) and for meeting any increase in the metabolism of the pregnant mother.

5.6.2   Requirements

The NE (E_c) requirements for pregnancy were described in Section 2.1.5 and tabulated in Table 2.8. Since the energy requirements of pregnancy are $1/0.133 = 7.5$ J of ME per J of NE of the conceptus (E_c) deposited per day, the resulting estimates of ME requirements above maintenance (M_c) for the last 3 months of pregnancy in dairy goats are given in Table 5.7.

Table 5.7: Additional metabolisable energy requirements (MJ ME/d) above maintenance for dairy goats in the last 3 months of pregnancy, assuming a requirement of 7.5 MJ ME/MJ energy deposited[1].

Month of pregnancy	Number of foetuses	Dairy goats			Fibre goats	
		1	2	3	1	2
3 (77 d)	Deposition[2]	0.11	0.18	0.25	0.07	0.10
	ME requirement	0.83	1.35	1.88	0.53	0.75
4 (105 d)	Deposition[2]	0.26	0.43	0.59	0.15	0.23
	ME requirement	1.95	3.23	4.43	1.13	1.73
5 (133 d)	Deposition[2]	0.49	0.82	1.09	0.29	0.44
	ME requirement	3.68	6.15	8.18	2.18	3.30

[1] Based on Table 2.7, and efficiency of utilisation of ME for the conceptus of 0.133 (ARC 1980).
[2] From Table 2.7.

5.7   Requirements for lactation and associated live-weight changes

5.7.1   Efficiency of ME utilisation

The estimation of efficiency of utilisation of ME for lactation (k_l) presents considerable difficulties as an increase in intake of ME during lactation results in a change in both milk production and the rate of deposition or mobilisation of energy in the body of the lactating female. There is, therefore, a need to estimate two efficiency terms for the lactating female:

(i) the efficiency of utilisation when the female's body is not changing in energy content (k_l).

The use of ME for milk secretion when no change in body energy is occurring is affected by the metabolisability (q_m) of the diet consumed, as shown in Table 5.1. The values for diets with metabolisabilities of 0.4 to 0.7

vary from 0.56 to 0.665. Aguilera *et al* (1990) found that the efficiency in lactating Granadina goats was slightly higher, by about 0.02 units, than the value predicted by the ARC (1980) equation for the diet used.

(ii) the efficiency with which body reserves are used for milk secretion when the intake of ME is less than the amount needed to achieve zero energy retention in the animal (k_t).

ARC (1980) gave an efficiency of utilisation of body energy for milk production (k_t) of 0.84.

5.7.2   Requirements

In Table 5.8, estimates of the ME requirements of 65-kg Anglo-Nubian and Saanen/Toggenburg goats for maintenance and the production of milk are given, using the ARC (1980) feeding level correction factor, C_L. No adjustments for net loss or gain of body energy are included.

Using the [EV_g] value of 23.9 MJ/kg live-weight adopted in Section 2.1.4.1, for a dietary q_m value of 0.6 ($k_l = 0.63$) goat dietary ME requirements in early lactation can be reduced by 31.9 MJ/kg live-weight loss. At an average live-weight loss of 1 kg/week in the first 4 weeks of lactation as suggested by INRA (1988), this amounts to 4.6 MJ ME/d, in reasonable agreement with the INRA recommended figure of 5.8 MJ ME/d (0.53 UFL/d). There seems good agreement that lactating goats can contribute the equivalent of 4 to 6 MJ ME daily in the first month of lactation. It is proposed here to adopt the ARC (1980) value of 4.6 MJ ME equivalent per day,

Table 5.8: Requirements for energy (MJ ME/d) during the lactation of 65-kg goats neither losing nor gaining body energy reserves.

Milk yield (kg/d)	Anglo-Nubian[2]			Saanen/Toggenburg[2]		
	Metabolisability of diet (q_m)			Metabolisability of diet (q_m)		
	0.5	0.6	0.7	0.5	0.6	0.7
(Maintenance)[1]	12.5	11.9	11.3	12.5	11.9	11.3
1	18.3	17.3	16.5	17.4	16.5	15.7
2	24.1	22.9	21.7	22.3	21.2	20.1
3	30.1	28.5	27.1	27.3	25.9	24.6
4	36.2	34.2	32.5	32.4	30.7	29.1
5	42.3	40.0	38.0	37.5	35.5	33.7
6	48.6	45.9	43.6	42.8	40.5	38.4

[1] Energy cost of 315 kJ/kg $W^{0.75}$ daily plus 10% for activity, 5 kJ/kg for standing for 12 h/d and 3.12 kJ/kg for 12 position changes/d.
[2] Energy value of milk as given in Table 2.10; total ME requirement calculated using feeding level correction of 1.8% per multiple of maintenance, as for cows in ARC (1980).

representing a nominal live-weight loss of 1.0 kg per week, which will be used to estimate the protein contribution also.

5.8. Requirements for gains in body energy in lactating goats

5.8.1 Efficiency of ME utilisation

A number of studies have shown that in lactating cows and goats the efficiency of utilisation of ME for body gain (k_g) is much higher than in non-lactating animals, and close to the efficiency of utilisation for milk secretion, k_l. ARC (1980), therefore, proposed that energy is deposited in the lactating ruminant with an efficiency of 0.95 k_l. Estimates in lactating goats of 0.964 k_l by Armstrong and Blaxter (1965) and of 0.974 k_l by Aguilera *et al* (1990) confirm that the general value of 0.95 k_l for lactating ruminants is likely to be correct for lactating goats.

5.8.2 Requirements

From the work of Dunshea *et al* (1990) a value of 23 MJ/kg live-weight gain in lactating goats can be calculated (see Section 2.1.4). This is close to the value of 23.9 MJ/kg live weight adopted above from ARC (1980). Taking the ARC (1980) value for efficiency of $0.95k_l$, a monthly gain of 1.2 kg (40 g/d) as recommended by INRA (1988) for multiparous goats would require 1.7 MJ ME/d. For primiparous goats INRA (1988) recommended a live-weight gain of 2.2 kg/month (73 g/d) which would require 2.9 MJ ME/d.

6.   Protein

For many years the basic unit for estimating the protein requirements of ruminants was digestible crude protein (DCP), and total protein and DCP were the units adopted by NRC (1981) in estimating the nutrient requirements of goats. However, progress in the 1960s in understanding and quantifying the processes of digestion and synthesis of protein in the rumen led to the realisation of the inadequacies of the DCP system. In the past 10 to 15 years many countries have introduced new systems based on predicting the supply of microbial and feed protein to the intestines, the digestion of protein and absorption of amino acids from the intestines, and the efficiency of utilisation of absorbed amino acids for maintenance and production. Although all of these systems are similar in concept, they differ in detail and continue to be subject to review and improvement. In France, recommendations for goats based on a new system were published in 1978 by INRA (INRA 1978) and were revised 10 years later (INRA 1988). In the UK, the first new system was proposed in full in 1980 (ARC 1980) and this was modified in 1984 (ARC 1984). A revised scheme with a number of modifications to ARC (1984) was published by AFRC (1992). Subsequently, an Advisory Manual was compiled to incorporate the AFRC (1990) and (1992) recommendations on the energy and protein requirements of ruminants (AFRC 1993). In the present report, estimates of the protein requirements of goats are based on the metabolisable protein system recommended in AFRC (1992), which should be consulted for full details of the scheme. Estimates measured in goats for various factors required for the ARC (1984) and AFRC (1992) schemes will be compared with the values recommended for cattle and sheep in those reports.

6.1   Energy supply for microbial protein synthesis in the rumen

In ARC (1984), the amount of energy available for microbial protein synthesis was defined in terms of the proportion of apparently digestible organic matter

(DOM) that is apparently digested in the rumen (DOMR). Values for DOMR/ DOM measured in goats that have been published are summarised in Table 6.1. There is a wide variation in the DOMR/DOM values, but they do not differ consistently from those in the large survey for sheep or cattle in ARC (1980). The value adopted in ARC (1984) was 0.65 for all diets for both cattle and sheep.

However, the parameter DOMR/DOM was not used in the AFRC (1992) protein system, and it was proposed that microbial protein synthesis should be related to the amount of potentially fermentable ME [FME] in the feed or diet. They took the proposal of ARC (1984) that DOM digested in the rumen should be corrected for supplementary fat, since fat yields little or no ATP for microbial synthesis in the rumen, and applied a correction [ME_{fat}] based on the gross energy of all lipids present in the feed or diet. They also adopted the concept proposed by INRA (1988), that fermented OM (FOM) should be corrected for the presence of the fermentation acids (acetic, propionic, butyric and lactic acids) arising from the microbial fermentation of feeds such as silage or brewers' grains. These organic acids, although a source of energy to the host animal, do not yield much ATP for microbial synthesis, since they are themselves the end products of microbial activity. The correction term [ME_{ferm}] is based on the GE values of the acids involved. The term [FME] is therefore defined as:

$$[FME] \text{ MJ/kg DM} = [ME] - [ME_{fat}] - [ME_{ferm}]$$

The adoption of this term rationalises the low microbial synthesis values variously reported on grass silages, which have only about 0.7, (varying 0.40

Table 6.1: Measurements of the proportion of digestible organic matter apparently digested in the rumen (DOMR/DOM) in goats.

Reference	Animals	Diets	Treatments	DOMR/DOM
Alam *et al* (1987)	4-month-old kids and lambs	High quality meadow hay	40 g OM/kg $W^{0.75}$ daily	0.69 (lambs 0.71)
			65 g OM/kg $W^{0.75}$ daily	0.74 (lambs 0.62)
Ash and Norton (1987a)	8-month-old cashmere goats	Straw/ concentrate pellets	113 g CP/kg DM	0.57
			213 g CP/kg DM	0.77
Kameoka and Morimoto (1959)	Adult goats	Forages only Mixed diets		0.75 to 0.85 0.62 to 0.82

to 0.85) of the silage [ME] present as [FME], and also explains the observed effects of supplementary fat in dairy cow diets.

6.2   Feed nitrogen degradability

In AFRC (1992) feed nitrogen is divided into three fractions: quickly degradable N [QDN], slowly degradable N [SDN] and undegradable N [UDN] based on their degradability in the rumen:

1. [QDN] is the fraction of total N washed out of the polyester bag when using the procedure of Ørskov and Mehrez (1977).
2. [SDN] is the amount of degradable N, other than [QDN] predicted to be available using the equation of Ørskov and McDonald (1979) for effective degradability (p), where rumen outflow rate (r/h) is taken into account.
3. [UDN] is the difference between total N and the sum of [QDN] and [SDN] at any given outflow rate.

Only Ash (1986) appears to have measured N degradability in goats *in vivo*. He obtained values of 0.78 and 0.89 for pelleted diets of straw/sorghum/ cotton seed meal containing 113 and 213 g CP/kg DM respectively. These values are high although within the very wide range of values for sheep (0.14 to 0.92) in ARC (1980).

A small number of estimates of effective degradabilities (degradability measured in polyester bags, adjusted for fractional outflow rates, r/h) have been published for goats. The values (Table 6.2) vary widely and do not lead to any clear conclusions regarding differences between goats and sheep and cattle. Hadjipanayiotou *et al* (1988b) found similar degradabilities in goats and sheep for soyabean meal and fishmeal at a maintenance level of feeding.

6.3   Apparent efficiency of conversion of degradable dietary nitrogen into microbial nitrogen

There appears to be no published information for goats. In AFRC (1992) the following values were adopted:

1. QDN: the recommendations of ARC (1984) of a value of 0.8 for the net efficiency of conversion of non-protein N fractions to microbial N have been adopted for the QDN fraction by AFRC (1992).
2. SDN: AFRC (1992) adopted the ARC (1980) recommendation that degradable protein is converted to microbial protein with a net efficiency of 1.0.

These two fractions, QDN and SDN are then combined with the adopted conversion efficiencies into a new parameter, effective rumen degradable N

Table 6.2: Estimates of effective protein degradability (p) in goats measured in synthetic fibre bags.

Reference	Principal concentrate constituents (g/kg)[1]	Fractional rumen outflow rate per hour (r)	Effective degradability (p)
Badamana (1987)	Barley 720	0.070	0.65
	Barley 635/SBM 105	0.075	0.60
	Barley 550/SBM 210	0.079	0.63
	Barley 720	0.070	0.64
	Barley 550/SBM 210	0.079	0.71
	Barley 380/SBM 425	0.082	0.71
Hadjipanayiotou *et al* (1988b)	Soyabean meal	0.050	0.28
	Fishmeal	0.050	0.39
Hadjipanayiotou *et al* (1988a)	Barley 736/SBM 195	0.050	0.45
	Barley 769/SBM 112/FM 50	0.050	0.46
	Barley 740/FM 121	0.050	0.38

[1]SBM = soyabean meal; FM = fishmeal.

(ERDN), as a measure of the N supply to the rumen microbes:

$$ERDN = 0.8QDN + SDN$$

The amount of ERDN converted to microbial crude protein (MCP) is dependent on energy (FME) supply with efficiencies as noted in Section 6.4.

6.4   Microbial nitrogen yield in the rumen

In ARC (1984) it was concluded that, for diets consisting of a well-balanced mixture of roughage and concentrates, or of fresh or dried high-quality grass and legume forage, a value of 32 g microbial nitrogen (MN)/kg DOMR should be adopted, equivalent to a value of 1.34 g MN/MJ ME (8.38 g MCP/ MJ ME. However, it was further suggested that there was some evidence to support different values for certain diets.

The values for the efficiency of MN synthesis in the rumen determined in goats given in Table 6.3 are within the ranges listed in ARC (1980) and (1984), though tending to be higher than the values adopted in ARC (1984). The results from Laurent *et al* (1987) were with lactating goats with duodenal cannulas and ribonucleic acid (RNA) was used as the microbial marker. Those of Ash and Norton (1987a) were with young feral kids with abomasal cannulas and ^{35}S was used as the marker. Reviews have been published

(Brun-Bellut *et al* 1987; Morand-Fehr *et al* 1987) of largely unpublished French results (including those of Laurent *et al* 1987), which were based on RNA flows at the duodenum of lactating goats given unspecified diets and on measurements of indigestible MN in the faeces and a regression analysis.

Table 6.3: Measurements of the efficiency of microbial crude protein (MCP, N × 6.25) synthesis in the rumen of goats.

Reference	Diet	Microbial crude protein synthesis		
		g MCP/kg DOM	g MN/kg DOMR[2]	g MCP/MJ ME[2]
Laurent *et al* (1987)	Hay, concentrates	109[1]		7.0
	Ryegrass, concentrates	161[1]		10.3
	Maize silage	159[1]		10.2
Ash and Norton (1987a)	113g CP/kg DM		46[1]	10.6
	213g CP/kg DM		36[1]	11.9
Brun-Bellut *et al* (1987)	Various	98 to 179[1]		6.3–11.5
Morand-Fehr *et al* (1987)	Various	150[1]		9.6

[1] Values published.
[2] Calculated assuming 1 kg DOM = 15.58 MJ ME and DOMR = 0.65 as ARC (1984).

Given that the ranges of the values for DOMR/DOM and MN/DOMR found for goats are similar to those for cattle and sheep, the proposals of AFRC (1992) for the microbial crude protein yield (y) as g/MJ of FME, where microbial N supply is not limiting, should be related to feeding level (L) are adopted here, namely:

At maintenance   (L = 1)   y = 9 g/MJ FME
At 2 times maintenance (L = 2), *c.* 3 kg milk/d, y = 10 g/MJ FME
At 3 times maintenance (L = 3), *c.* 6 kg milk/d, y = 11 g/MJ FME

When ERDP supply is not adequate to meet the amounts of MCP predicted by the functions suggested above, then it is assumed that microbial yield (MCP) will be equal to ERDP, irrespective of FME supply.

6.5 Proportion of microbial crude protein (MCP) present as microbial true protein (MTP)

There appears to be no published information on MTP/MCP for goats. A value of 0.80 was proposed in ARC (1984), reduced to 0.75 by AFRC (1992). The latter value is adopted for goats.

6.6 Absorbability of amino acids (AA) in the small intestine

In ARC (1980) a value for apparent absorbability of AA-N of 0.7 was adopted. This was based on mean values for various diets ranging from 0.64 to 0.67 for cattle and 0.63 to 0.73 for sheep. In ARC (1984) true absorbability replaced apparent absorbability and a value of 0.85 was adopted, whilst INRA (1988) assumed a value of 0.80. AFRC (1992) accepted the ARC (1984) value of 0.85 for the true absorption of MTP in the intestine.

There appear to be no estimates of the true absorbability of amino acids in goats although a few estimates of apparent absorption have been published. Alam *et al* (1987) obtained values for the apparent absorbability of non-ammonia N (NAN) between the abomasum and ileum of 0.64 and 0.65 for kids and lambs respectively at maintenance intakes, and 0.60 for both species at *ad libitum* intakes. Ash and Norton (1987a) estimated the apparent absorbability of NAN in the whole intestines to be 0.74 and 0.64 for diets containing 113 or 213 g CP/kg DM respectively.

These values are within the range for apparent absorption in sheep in ARC (1980) and it is suggested that it is appropriate to adopt the general value of 0.85 for true absorption of MTP in the intestine of goats.

6.7 Digestibility of undegraded feed protein

ARC (1980) and ARC (1984) assumed that the apparent digestibilities of MCP and undegraded feed protein (UDP) were the same, and assigned values of 0.7 and 0.85, respectively. However, ARC (1984) recognised that the fraction, acid detergent insoluble N [ADIN] might be a measure of the totally indigestible N fraction of feeds. AFRC (1992) adopted the function proposed by Webster *et al* (1984) for the prediction of the digestible undegraded N [UDN] of a feed or diet, based on [ADIN]:

$$[DUN] = 0.9([UDN] - [ADIN])$$

This gives a working range of about 0.4 to 0.85 for the digestibility of UDN. These proposals of AFRC (1992) for the digestibility of UDN are here adopted for goats.

The sum of DMTP and DUP supplied by a diet was defined as metabolisable protein supply (MPS) in AFRC (1992) and is equal to truly absorbed amino acid nitrogen (AA-N) $\times$ 6.25. The terms PDI in INRA (1988) and AAT of Madsen (1985) are similarly defined.

6.8   Efficiency of utilisation of absorbed amino acid nitrogen by ruminants

In ARC (1980) a value of 0.75 was proposed for the efficiency of utilisation of apparently absorbed AA-N (k_n) for all purposes. In ARC (1984), consequent on the decision to base maintenance requirements on total endogenous nitrogen (TEN), estimates of AA-N supply were changed to truly absorbed AA-N and a value of 0.80 was proposed for the efficiency of utilisation of "protein of good amino acid balance and under N-limiting conditions" for all purposes, including maintenance.

AFRC (1992) considered this topic in detail and proposed a value of 0.85 for k_{aai}, defined as "the efficiency with which a mixture of absorbed amino acids in ideal proportions is used for tissue protein or milk protein". AFRC (1992) also took the view that k_{aai} for the replenishment of basal endogenous losses of N (BEN, maintenance), will in effect be 1.0 under normal feeding circumstances, as this will be an obligatory demand on the available AA. AFRC (1992) further developed this concept by proposing the term "relative value" (RV) of the amino acid supplied as compared with the ideal mixture, and different efficiencies of utilisation for different processes. By combining values for k_{aai}, RV and efficiencies of utilisation, the following "working values" are proposed by AFRC (1992) for the efficiencies of utilisation of AA-N likely to be found in practice:

maintenance, k_{nm} 1.0
growth, k_{nf} 0.59
pregnancy, k_{nc} 0.85
lactation, k_{nl} 0.68
wool, k_{nw} 0.26

The concept of different efficiencies for different processes has already been adopted in the US (NRC 1985a), French (Vérité *et al* 1987), and Nordic (Madsen 1985) schemes. In the following sections, the available evidence for goats will be reviewed against this background.

6.9   Requirements for maintenance

Central to calculations of the efficiency of utilisation of absorbed amino acid-N (AA-N) is the definition of maintenance N requirements, basal (total) endogenous N (BEN, TEN), defined in Section 6.9.4.

6.9.1   Endogenous urinary nitrogen

Endogenous urinary N (EUN) is considered to represent the inevitable losses of N from the body associated with the maintenance of body function, particularly the breakdown and synthesis of protein. It can be estimated either by measuring N losses at very low N intakes or by regressing urinary N on some measure of N supply.

Published estimates for goats range widely, from 0.038 to 0.237 g N/kg $W^{0.75}$ daily (Table 6.4). The majority of values are in a much narrower range of 0.10 to 0.13 g N/kg $W^{0.75}$ daily. The greatest uncertainty concerns lactating goats. One group of French workers found almost identical values for lactating goats, 0.111 g N/kg $W^{0.75}$ daily (Brun-Bellut *et al* 1984) and castrated males, 0.113 g N/kg $W^{0.75}$ daily (Blanchart *et al* 1980). In contrast, a group of Spanish workers reported values to be 88% higher for lactating goats, 0.218 g N/kg $W^{0.75}$ daily (Aguilera *et al* 1990) than for castrated males of the same breed, 0.119 g N/kg $W^{0.75}$ daily (Prieto *et al* 1990). A value of 0.17 g N/kg $W^{0.75}$ daily for lactating goats determined by Giger (1987) is intermediate.

From these estimates a mean value of 0.12 g N/kg $W^{0.75}$ daily seems a reasonable estimate for EUN losses for non-lactating goats. Compared with values in ARC (1980) for sheep of the same weight, the resulting estimates of EUN losses for non-lactating goats are lower for animals weighing less than about 15 kg but higher for animals weighing more than 20 kg. For lactating goats no satisfactory value can be derived from published estimates and more experimental work is required. However, it should be noted that estimates of EUN in ARC (1980) do not distinguish between lactating and non-lactating stock for either cattle or sheep. The proposals of AFRC (1992), following ARC (1984), to adopt BEN as a measure of maintenance needs for N, include EUN within the requirement for BEN.

6.9.2   Metabolic faecal nitrogen

Metabolic faecal N (MFN) is generally considered to represent the N in the faeces of animals given N-free diets. It can be determined by methods similar to those used for calculating EUN. In practice, reliable values are difficult to obtain. The earlier view that MFN is largely endogenous in origin has been challenged by findings indicating that a high proportion is microbial (Mason 1969). It has been considered to be both endogenous (ARC 1965) and exogenous (ARC

1980), depending on the model being adopted to describe N transactions.

In attempts to predict MFN losses, faecal N excretion has most commonly been related to DM intake. Published values are relatively few and, with one exception, are in the range 4 to 5 g N/kg DM intake (Table 6.4), equivalent to about 0.15 to 0.20 g N/kg $W^{0.75}$ daily. Maintenance MFN losses are included within the stated requirement for BEN of AFRC (1992) of 0.35 g N/kg $W^{0.75}$ daily.

6.9.3   Dermal losses

There appear to be no direct estimates of N losses in hair and scurf (N_d) by non-fibre goats. A value of 0.018 g N/kg $W^{0.75}$ daily was adopted by ARC (1980) for cattle. Morand-Fehr *et al* (1987) have proposed that a value of 0.02 g N/kg $W^{0.75}$ daily, also based on cattle, should be used for goats. The ARC (1980) estimate of 0.018 g N/kg $W^{0.75}$ daily, (0.113 g NP_d/kg $W^{0.75}$ daily) for cattle is adopted for goats here. Dermal losses are not included within BEN as proposed by AFRC (1992).

Table 6.4: Published estimates of endogenous urinary nitrogen (EUN), metabolic faecal nitrogen (MFN) and minimal nitrogen (N) losses in goats.

Reference	Animals	EUN (g/kg $W^{0.75}$ per day)	MFN (g/kg DM)	Minimal N losses (g/kg $W^{0.75}$ per day)
Majumdar (1960a)	Dry females	0.13	4.1	
Akinsoyinu *et al* (1975)	Dry females			0.273 to 0.393
Akinsoyinu *et al* (1976)	Dry females	0.038	4.3	
Itoh *et al* (1978)	Castrated males	0.237		
Blanchart *et al* (1980)	Castrated males	0.113		
Devendra (1980)	Dry females	0.133		
Rajpoot *et al* (1980)	Castrated males	0.105 to 0.115	4.3	
Reynolds (1981)	Castrated males	0.121	4.9	
Guerrero (1982)	Castrated males	0.123		
Brun-Bellut *et al* (1984)	Lactating	0.111	1.1	
Ciszuk and Lindberg (1985)	Lactating[1] (a)			0.229
	(b)			0.127
Giger (1987)	Lactating	0.17		
Prieto *et al* (1990)	Castrated males	0.119		0.108
Aguilera *et al* (1990)	Lactating	0.218		0.244
Alam *et al* (1991)	4-month-old kids			0.296 to 0.334

[1] (a) Calculated by the authors at zero digestible organic matter intake.
   (b) Calculated at zero truly absorbed amino acid N from authors' regression equation.

6.9.4   Total endogenous nitrogen or basal endogenous nitrogen

If TEN is considered to represent the sum of EUN, MFN and dermal losses, values between about 0.25 and 0.35 g N/kg $W^{0.75}$ daily are obtained from the mean values in the preceding sections. When N balance is regressed against a measure of N supply, the negative intercept at zero N intake provides an estimate of minimum N losses which should be similar to the sum of EUN and MFN (Table 6.4). Aguilera *et al* (1990) have recently calculated a value of 0.244 g N/kg $W^{0.75}$ daily for lactating Granadina goats at zero N intake but losses of only 0.108 g N/kg $W^{0.75}$ daily were found by the same group (Prieto *et al* 1990) for castrated male goats. Ciszuk and Lindberg (1985) proposed a value of 0.229 g N/kg $W^{0.75}$ daily for lactating Swedish Landrace goats, which is close to that of Aguilera *et al* (1990). However, this value was calculated at zero OM intake, not at zero N intake. When the results are related to truly absorbed AA-N, the estimate of minimal N losses at zero AA-N uptake becomes 0.127 g N/kg $W^{0.75}$ daily.

Working with 4-month-old lambs and feral kids, Alam *et al* (1991) calculated values of 0.296 to 0.334 g N/kg $W^{0.75}$ daily for the kids, which weighed about 14 kg, but only 0.198 to 0.234 g N/kg $W^{0.75}$ daily for the lambs, which weighed about 23 kg; both were determined at zero apparent digestion of amino acids in the intestine.

These published values vary widely and almost all are below the value of 0.35 g N/kg $W^{0.75}$ daily proposed for cattle and sheep in ARC (1984) on the basis of a different experimental approach.

ARC (1984) argued that part of the fraction conventionally measured as MFN was a component of total endogenous N (TEN) losses which therefore consisted of EUN, part of MFN and dermal losses. It was further argued that the only method available for measuring TEN losses was based on the intra-gastric infusion technique (Ørskov *et al* 1979). On the basis of a small number of measurements using this technique with cattle and sheep, a value for 350 mg N/kg $W^{0.75}$ daily was proposed for TEN. This value has subsequently been accepted by AFRC (1992) but renaming TEN as the BEN requirement of ruminants, which is the term used here. In terms of net protein (NP), the term BEN becomes 2.19 g NP_b/kg $W^{0.75}$ daily.

6.9.5   Efficiency of AA utilisation for maintenance

There appear to be no experimental results with goats to relate directly to recently proposed values for k_{nm} (ARC 1984; AFRC 1992). The majority of published estimates are based on the efficiency of utilisation of apparently digestible CP (digestible N) which cannot readily be converted to truly absorbed AA-N. Indeed, Ciszuk and Lindberg (1985) showed that when such widely divergent N sources as urea and fishmeal were compared for lactating goats the efficiencies, based on digestible N and on AA-N, were widely different.

Using regression analysis of the results of N-balance studies with lactating goats, Brun-Bellut *et al* (1984) calculated that the efficiency of utilisation of apparently digestible N for maintenance (k_{nm}) was 0.78. From results of these and other largely unpublished French experiments with lactating goats, Morand-Fehr *et al* (1987) calculated an efficiency for the utilisation of truly absorbed AA-N of 0.83. Although these findings support the original recommendation of 0.85 by ARC (1984), we accept the arguments of AFRC (1992) for the higher value of 1.0 for k_{nm}.

6.9.6   Requirements

Published values for goats vary widely but there is no compelling evidence that maintenance requirements differ appreciably from those for cattle and sheep. On the basis of AFRC (1992) proposals for BEN losses of 0.35 g N/kg $W^{0.75}$ daily and an efficiency of utilisation of 1.0, the maintenance requirement for goats is 0.35 g truly absorbed AA-N/kg $W^{0.75}$ daily (2.19 g MP_m/kg $W^{0.75}$ daily).

6.10   Requirements for lactation

6.10.1   Efficiency of AA utilisation for lactation

Brun-Bellut *et al* (1984) calculated the efficiency of converting digestible N to milk N to be 0.72 to 0.81 in lactating goats given a variety of diets, though in N-deficient goats the efficiency was only 0.56. Calculating efficiency as milk N/(digestible N − maintenance N), Brun-Bellut *et al* (1987) found values ranging from 0.31 to 0.75 from various published reports. Morand-Fehr *et al* (1987) reported that the efficiency of using predicted truly absorbed AA-N for milk N (k_{nl}) was 0.80 for diets rich in fermentable N (Giger 1987) and 0.75 for diets deficient in fermentable N (Brun-Bellut 1986). Ciszuk and Lindberg (1985) calculated the efficiencies of using digestible N and truly absorbed AA-N for milk N and maintenance combined were 0.54 and 0.71 respectively at peak lactation. In mid-lactation, respective values were 0.65 and 0.75 for low-N diets, but these fell with increasing N content in the diet.

Morand-Fehr *et al* (1987) concluded that the efficiencies of producing milk N from truly absorbed AA-N in excess of maintenance requirements found for goats are in the same range as those reported for dairy cows (Vérité *et al* 1987). They recommended that the same value, 0.64, be used for the two species, which is very similar to the value of 0.68 for k_{nl} recommended by AFRC (1992). These recommended values are lower than the highest experimental values but probably represent the best estimates available for use in practical feeding conditions.

It is recommended that the value of 0.68 for the conversion of truly absorbed AA-N to milk AA-N (k_{nl}) should be adopted for lactating goats.

6.10.2   *Efficiency of utilisation of mobilised body protein for lactation*

Dairy goats mobilise body protein in early lactation (Brun-Bellut *et al* 1984) and deposit it later in lactation but little is known about the extent or efficiency of either process. ARC (1980) implied an efficiency of mobilisation of body tissue protein AA of 1.0, since they adopted an efficiency of utilisation of 0.75 for mobilised body tissue protein, identical to that for absorbed AA. This efficiency coefficient of 1.0 has also been adopted by AFRC (1992) for lactating goats, the mobilised amino acids then being used with an efficiency of 0.68 for the synthesis of milk protein. Brun-Bellut *et al* (1984) calculated that the efficiency of converting body N to milk N was 0.71, close to the AFRC (1992) value of 0.68.

6.10.3   *Requirements*

ARC (1984) calculated the RDP and UDP requirements of lactating cattle and sheep from the total AA-N content of milk (equivalent to the true protein content/6.38), and AFRC (1992) continued this when calculating the [NP_l] content of milk and the MP requirements of lactating ruminants. The true protein content [NP_l] of goats' milk was defined in 2.11.2 of this report as 0.9 times the CP content [CP].

On the basis of a value of 0.68 for k_{nl} for the conversion of truly absorbed AA-N to milk AA-N, the requirement for the production of 1 kg milk is estimated to be 7.6 g truly absorbed AA-N (47.7 g MP) for the Anglo-Nubian group (36 g crude protein/kg; Table 2.11) and 6.1 g truly absorbed AA-N (38.4 g MP) for the Saanen/Toggenburg group (29 g CP/kg; Table 2.11). The very limited evidence available (Table 2.10) suggests that AA-N requirements for milk synthesis for lactating feral cashmere goats may be similar to those of Anglo-Nubians. The MP requirements of lactating goats in early and mid lactation are given later in Section 6.14, Table 6.7.

6.11   Requirements for growth

6.11.1   *Efficiency of AA utilisation for growth*

Comparing growth in 4-month-old kids and lambs, Alam *et al* (1991) calculated that the efficiency of converting apparently absorbed AA-N to pelage-free body N (k_{nf}) was 0.52 in the kids and 0.29 in the lambs. Equivalent efficiencies in body plus pelage were 0.50 and 0.41 respectively. In the absence of direct experimental evidence for goats, Morand-Fehr *et al*

(1987) recommended the use of an efficiency of 0.65 for the utilisation of truly absorbed AA-N in young kids, which was a figure based on values for cattle reducing from 0.68 to 0.40 with increasing age (Vérité *et al* 1987). A value of 0.59 for k_{nf} for growth in ruminants is recommended by AFRC (1992) and it is recommended that this value should be adopted for goats.

6.11.2 Requirements

Table 6.5 gives the requirements for truly absorbed AA-N (g/d) for growth, calculated on the basis of an efficiency of utilisation of truly absorbed AA-N (k_{nf}) of 0.59 and protein deposition in growing kids as in Table 2.4.

Table 6.5: Requirements for truly absorbed amino acids (metabolisable protein, MP_f) for the growth of goat kids.

Body weight growth interval	MP$_f$ requirements (g/d)		
	15–20 kg	20–25 kg	25–30 kg
Rate of growth			
100 g/d	24.6	24.0	23.4
200 g/d	49.2	48.0	46.8
300 g/d	73.8	72.0	70.2

Note: Based on equation in Table 2.4: $NP_f = 157.22 - 0.694W$ and $k_{ng} = 0.59$.

6.12   Requirements for fibre

There is little information about the protein requirements for fibre production in goats. Mohair production by Angora goats has been found to be depressed by low protein levels in the diet (Van der Westhuysen *et al*, 1985). NRC (1981) recommended 3 g DCP/d for every kg fleece produced annually, which INRA (1988) equated to 2.5 g PDI/d/kg fleece. For a typical 7-kg mohair fleece, this results in a 0.35 increase in maintenance protein requirements expressed as PDI. Norton and Ash (1985) reviewed the protein requirements for cashmere (guard hair plus down) production in goats and quoted experiments where cashmere production was unresponsive to protein supply. They concluded that the protein requirements for cashmere production are probably very low, because the goat only produces small amounts of cashmere (50–500 g). They also calculated that less than 0.01 of dietary protein intake is required to grow a cashmere fleece compared with 0.06 to

0.09 in sheep. It is possible that the maximum protein requirements for cashmere are met in all but the severest nutritional crisis.

6.12.1   *Efficiency of AA utilisation for fibre growth*

There appears to be no experimental evidence concerning the efficiency of N utilisation for fibre production by goats. SCA (1990), after reviewing the published work on wool fibre production and concluding that low efficiencies of utilisation of the order of 0.2 had been recorded, chose to adopt a value of 0.6, on the grounds that it was unlikely that sheep would waste 0.8 of the AA-N not utilised for wool synthesis. Assuming an RV of 0.3, a value of 0.26 was proposed by AFRC (1992) for the efficiency of utilisation of truly absorbed AA-N for wool growth (k_{nw}) and it is recommended, in the absence of any experimental evidence for goats, that this value be adopted for fibre production by goats.

6.12.2   *Requirements*

Based on an efficiency of utilisation (k_{nw}) of 0.26 and the nutrient retentions in goat fibre given in Table 2.16, requirements for truly absorbed AA-N are 6.2 g/d (38.5 g MP/d) for Angora goats and 2.2 g/d (13.6 g MP/d), from June to December only, for cashmere goats.

6.13   Requirements for pregnancy

6.13.1   *Efficiency of AA utilisation for pregnancy*

There appears to be no experimental evidence concerning the efficiency of N utilisation for pregnancy (k_{nc}) in goats. A value of 0.85 for ruminants is proposed by AFRC (1992) and it is recommended that this value be adopted for goats.

6.13.2   *Requirements*

Table 6.6 gives requirements for pregnancy on the basis of the estimated protein deposition (NP_c) in the gravid uterus of either dairy and fibre goats with single, twin or triplet kids as tabulated in Table 2.8, and using an efficiency of truly absorbed AA-N utilisation (k_{nc}) of 0.85.

Table 6.6: Additional requirements of dairy and fibre goats for truly absorbed amino acids (metabolisable protein, MP_c) during the last 3 months of pregnancy.

Weeks before parturition	Weeks pregnant	Dairy (D) or fibre (F)	MP_c requirements (g/d)		
			Singles	Twins	Triplets
12–8	9–13	D	4.4	7.2	10.0
		F	2.8	4.2	–
8–4	13–17	D	10.1	17.2	23.5
		F	6.1	9.5	–
4–0	17–term	D	19.2	32.2	43.2
		F	11.6	17.9	–

Note: MP_c values are (1/0.85) times protein depositions (NP_c) in Table 2.8.

Table 6.7: Metabolisable protein requirements (MP, g/d) of lactating, multiparous, 65-kg Anglo-Nubian and Saanen/Toggenburg dairy goats.

Daily milk yield, kg/d	Anglo-Nubian			Saanen/Toggenburg		
	Month 1[1]	Months 2–3	Months 4–9[2]	Month 1[1]	Months 2–3	Months 4–9[2]
1	70	100	104	61	91	95
2	118	148	152	99	129	133
3	166	196	200	138	168	172
4	213	243	247	176	206	210
5	261	291	295	215	245	249
6	309	339	343	253	283	287

[1] A deficit of 30 g MP/d is accepted in month 1 of lactation.
[2] Assuming live-weight gain of 1.2 kg/month, equivalent to 4 g MP/d. For primiparous goats, a further 9 g/d should be added to allow for a growth rate of 2.2 kg/month.

6.14 Requirements for live-weight change in lactating goats

6.14.1 Mobilisation of body protein in early lactation

On the basis of feeding trials, INRA (1988) found it necessary for the protein requirements of lactating goats to be totally covered by the third week of lactation. They suggested that a maximum deficit of 85 g and 25 g PDI/d (equivalent to 51 g and 15 g NP_g/d) can be tolerated in the first and second weeks of lactation, respectively. This is apparently associated with a live-weight loss of 1 kg per week. Accordingly it is suggested that MP allowances for lactating goats may be reduced by 30 g MP/d, a total of 900 g MP in the first month of lactation, which for the nominal 1.0 kg live-weight loss per week allowed for energy, implies an NP_g for live-weight loss of 143 g/kg, comparable to the ARC (1980) recommendation of 119 g/kg for ewes and 138 g/kg for cows.

6.14.2   Live-weight gain in lactating goats

INRA (1988) recommended 4 g PDI/d and 13 g PDI/d for live-weight gains of 1.2 kg/month (40 g/d) for multiparous and 2.2 kg/month (73 g/d) for primiparous goats respectively. Using the ARC (1980) values for live-weight gain in ewes of 83 g NPg/kg, and the AFRC (1993) value for efficiency of MP utilisation, k_{ng} of 0.59, gives an MP requirement of 5.6 g/d, slightly higher than that recommended by INRA (1988) for multiparous goats. The INRA (1988) recommendations are adopted here, but expressed as metabolisable protein, ie 4 g MP/d for multiparous goats and 13 g MP/d for primiparous goats from the fourth month of lactation onwards for live-weight gains of 40 g/d and 73 g/d respectively.

The MP requirements of lactating Anglo-Nubian and Saanen/Toggenburg goats in early and mid lactation are given Table 6.7.

7.   Minerals and Vitamins

Published data on the mineral and vitamin content of the body tissues, blood and milk of goats are sparse (see Section 2), and there are relatively few scientific reports on other aspects of mineral and vitamin nutrition and metabolism which are of use in establishing requirements in this species. Reviews of goat mineral and vitamin nutrition, in general, provide little more than speculation based largely on analogy with cattle and sheep (e.g. Haenlein 1980b, 1984, 1987; Kessler 1981; Lamand 1981).

NRC (1981) based their recommendations for goats on sheep and cattle data, whilst those of Morand-Fehr *et al* (1987) and Morand-Fehr and Sauvant (1988) were also based largely on those for cattle and sheep, although data from feeding trials on the Ca and P contents of goats' milk and coefficients of absorption of Ca and P by goats were included. There is little information available on the basis for the recommendations of Eriksson *et al* (1976) or Skjevdal (1982). Those of Kessler (1984) are based mainly on INRA (1978) recommendations, with occasional unexplained modifications, whilst Kearl (1982) is largely based on NRC (1981) and Kessler (1981). In the UK, there are no official published values for the mineral and vitamin requirements of goats and recommendations are based on feeding standards from other countries, or they are extrapolated from the requirements of cattle and sheep.

Requirements for major minerals and some trace elements and vitamins were reviewed by ARC (1965) for sheep and cattle and updated by ARC (1980). Subsequently, an Inter-Departmental Working Party (IDWP), representing advisory, veterinary and feed industry interests, was established to assess whether or not it would be practicable to convert the ARC (1980) estimates of requirements into allowances (IDWP 1984). With a few exceptions, the IDWP (1984) recommendations supported the views of ARC (1980). There were large differences, however, between the recommended requirements for Ca and P proposed by ARC (1965) and those proposed by ARC (1980), and the IDWP (1984) decided to reject the proposals of ARC (1980) and to accept ARC (1965) values as dietary allowances. Subsequently, the AFRC Technical Committee on Responses to Nutrients (TCORN) set up a working party to assess the most recent research data relevant to the Ca and P requirements of ruminants, but their report (AFRC 1991) excluded any consideration of the Ca and P requirements of goats.

The present report compares feeding standards for goats published in other countries with estimated requirements for goats extrapolated from cattle and sheep recommendations put forward by ARC (1980), IDWP (1984) and AFRC (1991). It should be noted that the proposed requirements for goats are generalisations, and their application to specific breeds and conditions may vary.

7.1 Mineral composition of body tissues, milk and fibre

Knowledge of the mineral content of the goat body and products is essential if a factorial approach to the calculation of mineral requirements is adopted. From the reviews of body, milk and fibre composition (Sections 2.1, 2 and 3 respectively), it is concluded that limited data are available on milk composition but there is no specific information on the mineral content of the body tissues and fibre of goats.

It is suggested that the sheep values given by ARC (1980) for the mineral composition of the foetus, adnexa and newborn lambs should be adopted for the goat. The most appropriate model to use for the composition of live-weight gain in the growing animal is more questionable. For Ca and P, in particular, this is important as requirements are dominated by skeletal growth. Although lambs and calves have similar Ca and P contents, growing cattle appear to have a greater proportion of their live-weight gain as skeleton than do sheep, and this is responsible for the greater Ca and P content per unit growth in cattle compared to sheep (e.g. ARC 1980). In general, goats appear closer to cattle than to sheep in this respect. For example, Wood (1984) showed bone in the goat carcase to be 19% of the total carcase weight compared with 14% for the sheep carcase. This does not necessarily mean a higher proportion of bone in the whole body, but when correction is made for the greater amount of non-carcase fat in the goat the relative percentages of bone are still higher for the goat than for the sheep (16 and 13% respectively). Thus, in the absence of more reliable information on the Ca and P content of body weight gain in the goat, it seems prudent to base requirements for these minerals on the higher values found in cattle, but adjusted for the lower mature body weight (W_m) of goats, taken as 100 kg.

It is proposed that mineral requirements for fibre growth in goats should, at present, be based on the composition of the fleece of sheep. As for sheep, Ca, P and Mg requirements for fibre production are likely to be very low compared to those for maintenance, growth and milk production.

There is a some published information on Ca, P and Mg concentrations in goats' milk (Table 2.12) but for trace minerals, appropriate data on cows' milk will be used.

7.2   Calcium and phosphorus

7.2.1   *Metabolism*

In most respects Ca and P metabolism in goats appear to be similar to that in cattle and sheep (Haenlein 1980b, Hines *et al* 1986a, b). Near parturition, changes in blood Ca and P concentrations have been reported to be more similar to those in cattle than in sheep (Haenlein 1980b).

Although hypocalcaemia (milk fever) has been reported in goats (Haenlein 1987), the evidence from general observation (Haenlein 1984; Mowlem *pers comm*) is that goats are less susceptible to this disorder than cattle at comparable levels of production. This may be due to differences in hormonal responses during the period of high Ca demand following lactation, or to differences in the Ca content of typical rations fed to goats compared to cows, or to the level and/or type of stress imposed around parturition. Differences appear to exist between cattle and sheep in the timing of hypocalcaemia (Sykes and Russel 1991) and there may also be differences between goats and other ruminants, or even between types of goats in the manifestation or otherwise of hypocalcaemia.

7.2.2   *Systems for estimating Ca and P requirements*

Values for the parameters used in the factorial approaches to the estimation of the Ca and P requirements of goats are given in Table 7.1 for ARC (1980), IDWP (1984), INRA (1988) and AFRC (1991), but excluding NRC (1981), where the method of calculation is not given in the publication. They show differences not only in absolute terms, but in the fact that some systems use fixed values while others use ranges of values. The position is further complicated by differences in the criteria used to choose from such ranges (see footnotes to Table 7.1). Since the IDWP (1984) recommendations were based entirely on ARC (1965), they will not be considered further.

7.2.3   *Factors used by ARC (1980), AFRC (1991) and INRA (1988) to estimate Ca and P requirements*

(a)   *Endogenous loss of Ca*
ARC (1980) and INRA (1988) assumed similar and fixed values for endogenous losses of Ca. AFRC (1991) argued and produced convincing evidence for a range of values encompassing these, depending upon DM intake (DMI). It is proposed that the principle of AFRC (1991) for sheep should be adopted for the goat.

Table 7.1: Factors used in the different systems to estimate calcium and phosphorus requirements.

		Calcium				Phosphorus			
		ARC (1980)	IDWP (1984)	INRA (1988)	AFRC (1991)	ARC (1980)	IDWP (1984)	INRA (1988)	AFRC (1991)
Endogenous loss (mg/kg W daily)	Cattle	16	16	18	$10-25^2$	12	$14-30^1$	25	$9-35^2$
	Sheep	16	40	18	$14-35^2$	14	43.5	25	$12-40^2$
Composition of gain (g/kg LWG)	Cattle	14	$10.4-15.7^3$	$10-15^3$	$10.9-16.2^3$	8	$4.8-9.6^3$	$5-8^3$	$6.3-8.8^3$
	Sheep	11	8.9	$10-15^{3.5}$	$8.2-12.9^3$	6	5.0	$5-8^{3.5}$	$5.1-7.3^3$
True availability (fractional)	Cattle	0.68	$0.45-0.55^3$	$0.3-0.7^3$	0.68	$0.58-0.78^3$	$0.55-0.84^3$	$0.5-0.8^3$	$0.58-0.70^4$
	Sheep	0.68	$0.45-0.55^3$	$0.3-0.5^3$	0.68	$0.60-0.73^3$	$0.60-0.90^3$	$0.6-0.8^3$	$0.64-0.70^4$

[1] Increasing with age/maturity.
[2] Increasing with feed intake.
[3] Decreasing with age/maturity.
[4] Decreasing with high forage intakes.
[5] Values for sheep are considered to be slightly less than for cattle.

(b)   Endogenous loss of P

ARC (1980) assumed that endogenous losses of P were shown by loss of P on P-free diets. INRA (1988) did not accept this and adopted a much higher figure for endogenous losses. Once again, AFRC (1991) provided convincing new evidence for a range of values depending upon DMI, which encompassed both the low fixed ARC (1980) value and the high fixed INRA (1988) value. It is proposed that the principle of AFRC (1991) for the sheep be adopted for the goat.

(c)   Composition of gain

There is no direct information available on the Ca or P content of the whole body of the goat, although total ash data are available (Treacher *et al* 1987, Gibb *et al* 1993). It is proposed to adopt for goats the values given by ARC (1980) for cattle. ARC (1980) assumed a constant composition of Ca and P in the body of cattle irrespective of age. Both INRA (1988) and AFRC (1991) recognised that the proportion of skeletal mass decreases with age and proposed closely similar ranges of values for Ca and P in body-weight gain, dependent upon age and/or live weight. This principle, and values for cattle, are accepted for the goat.

(d)   Requirements for pregnancy

Requirements for pregnancy depend upon the size and number of kids produced. Values for the components of the gravid uterus in pregnant goats were calculated using the Gompertz functions and data for lowland ewes given in Robinson *et al* (1977), and McDonald *et al* (1979) as recommended in Section 2.1.5. Values for one, two or three foetuses at term for dairy and fibre producing goats in the fourth and fifth month of pregnancy were calculated.

(e)   Composition of milk

It is proposed that for general purposes mean values of 1.3 g Ca/kg and 0.9g P/kg (see Table 2.14) be used for milk from Saanen-type dairy breeds of goat. If compositional variations are known, actual values for milk composition should be used to calculate requirements.

(f)   True availability of Ca

Differences between sheep and cattle are very small for any of the systems, and it is proposed to use sheep values for the goat. There is a fundamental difference between INRA (1988) on the one hand, and ARC (1980) and AFRC (1991) on the other. ARC (1980) argued that as long as Ca is not given in excess it is always absorbed with a reasonably constant and high efficiency. AFRC (1991) took the same view and proposed the same fixed absorption coefficient as ARC (1980) (i.e. 0.68). INRA (1988), however, considered that the efficiency of absorption fell greatly in mature animals, for which they proposed a value of 0.3, which is responsible for the big differences in predicted requirements in mature animals and, indeed, explains many of the discrepancies between requirements proposed by INRA (1988) and the other systems.

The choice of absorption coefficient may be a rather subjective decision, but it is proposed that for the goat a value of 0.55 is adopted, as recommended by ARC (1965), to give a margin of safety, at least for the mature animal. It is important that excess Ca should not be given before parturition.

(g)   True availability of P
Reported differences between sheep and cattle are very small and it is proposed that sheep values be used for the goat. All systems proposed ranges of values between about 0.6 and 0.8, but ARC (1980) and INRA (1988) both assumed a decrease with maturity of the animal, while AFRC (1991) related lower values to high-roughage diets. The AFRC (1991) evidence seems sound and it is suggested that this principle should be adopted for goats.

7.2.4   Recommended dietary allowances of Ca and P for goats

The AFRC (1991) scheme, which forms the basis of the present recommendations, relates maintenance needs for both Ca and P to DMI. Thus requirements for Ca and P vary with the ME concentration in the diet, (q_m).

The estimated requirements for Ca and P given in Tables 7.2 to 7.5 (at metabolisability values (q_m) for appropriate diets) have been calculated based on the following considerations:

1. Endogenous loss (mg/kg live weight) for Ca and P is related to DMI according to the sheep equations in AFRC (1991), with the value for P multiplied by a factor of 1.6 for high forage diets ($q_m<0.7$; AFRC 1991).
2. The composition of gain (g/kg live weight), in terms of Ca and P for goats, is taken from the cattle composition data given by AFRC (1991), using a mature body weight of 65 kg for the female goat and 100 kg for the male.
3. Milk composition is assumed to be 1.3 g Ca and 0.9 g P/kg milk.
4. The true availability of dietary Ca is taken as 0.55 resulting in slightly higher estimates than those of AFRC (1991).
5. The true availability of P is taken as 0.64 for forage-based diets ($q_m<0.7$) and 0.7 for mainly cereal diets ($q_m = 0.7$ or greater).
6. Pregnancy needs for dairy goats are calculated from data given in ARC (1980) for ewes producing 3.95-kg twin lambs, or 3.65-kg triplets. The birth weights of cashmere kids are assumed to be either 2.75 kg for a single kid or 2.25 kg for twins.

Table 7.2: Predicted daily requirements (g/d) for calcium and phosphorus.

	IDWP (1984) (= ARC 1965)[1]		NRC (1981)[2]		ARC (1980)[1]		INRA (1988)		AFRC (1991)[1]		Present recommendations	
	Ca	P	Ca	P	Ca	P	Ca	P	Ca	P	Ca	P
Maintenance: 50-kg animal DMI = 2% body weight ($q_m < 0.7$)	4.5	2.7	4.0	2.8	1.2	1.2	3.5	2.5	1.3	1.6	1.6	1.6
Early lactation: 60-kg Saanen/Toggenburg animal yielding 5 kg milk/d DMI = 5% body weight ($q_m < 0.7$)	20	12	14	9.8	11	8.9	21.5	10	13	12	15.6	12.1
Late pregnancy, (week 16): 60-kg animal carrying 2 × 4.0 kg kids DMI = 2.5% body weight ($q_m < 0.7$)	9.2	6.1	6.0*	4.2*	4.8	3.1	10.0*	4.5*	5.1	4.0	4.6	3.7
Young male: 20-kg animal growing at 200 g/d DMI = 4.5% body weight ($q_m = 0.7$)	7.3	3.2	4.5	2.8	4.6	2.6	5.0	2.3	6.0	4.2	6.5	3.0
Young female: 30-kg animal growing at 100 g/d DMI = 2.5% body weight ($q_m < 0.7$)	5.2	2.7	3	2.1	2.8	1.7	4.4	2.0	3.4	2.5	3.4	2.2

* Values from published tables for late pregnancy; no details given of size or number of foetuses.
[1] Maintenance and pregnancy requirements based on sheep values; live-weight gain requirements on cattle values; lactation values based on goat milk composition. Young female assumed to be 6 to 12 months old; young male assumed to be < 6 months; 50-kg animal assumed to be 1 to 2 years old.
[2] Assuming maintenance plus appropriate growth/secretion.

Table 7.3: Dietary allowances of calcium and phosphorus (g/d) for growing goats.

Live weight (kg)	Dietary energy concentration (q_m)	Growth rate (g/d)					Growth rate (g/d)				
		0	50	100	150	200	0	50	100	150	200
		Ca requirement (g/d)					P requirement (g/d)				
10	0.7	–	2.2	3.7	5.3	6.9	–	0.8	1.5	2.2	2.8
20	0.7	–	2.2	3.5	4.9	6.3	–	0.9	1.5	2.2	2.8
30	0.6	1.1	2.4	3.7	5.0	6.4	0.9	1.6	2.4	3.3	4.1
40	0.5	1.5	2.8	4.1	5.5	–	1.5	2.3	3.3	4.3	–
60	0.5	1.9	3.2	4.5	–	–	2.1	3.0	4.1	–	–
80	0.5	2.2	3.6	–	–	–	2.6	3.7	–	–	–
100	0.5	2.6	–	–	–	–	3.1	–	–	–	–

Table 7.4: Dietary allowances of calcium and phosphorus (g/d) for maintenance and pregnancy of dairy and fibre goats.

Non-pregnant live weight (kg)	Dietary ME/GE (q_m)	Number of kids expected	Total weight of kids at term (kg)	Stage of gestation					
				Week 12		Week 16		Week 20	
				Requirement (g/d)					
				Ca	P	Ca	P	Ca	P
65		1	4.0	2.1	2.1	3.1	2.7	4.5	3.3
(Dairy goat)	0.60	2	7.95	2.6	2.5	4.6	3.6	7.3	4.8
		3	10.95	2.9	2.9	5.7	4.3	9.5	6.0
40		1	2.75	1.8	1.8	2.5	2.2	3.5	2.6
(Fibre goat)	0.50	2	4.5	2.0	2.0	3.2	2.6	4.8	3.4

7.3   Magnesium

7.3.1   Metabolism

Metabolism of Mg in the goat appears to be similar to that in other ruminants. Absorption is depressed by K although interactions between Mg and K may differ slightly from those observed with sheep (Haenlein 1980b, 1987). Magnesium deficiency (hypomagnesaemia) in the goat can cause tetany and hyper-irritability, while excess Mg may depress Ca absorption.

Table 7.5: Dietary allowances of calcium and phosphorus (g/d) for maintenance and during the lactation of 65-kg live weight Anglo-Nubian (A-N) and Saanen/Toggenburg (S/T) dairy goats.

Stage of lactation	Metabolisability of diet (q_m)	Breed of goat	Milk production (kg/d)											
			Ca requirement (g/d)						P requirement (g/d)					
			1	2	3	4	5	6	1	2	3	4	5	6
Early and mid	0.6	A-N	5.1	8.6	12.1	15.6	19.1	22.6	4.8	7.8	10.9	14.0	17.1	20.2
		S/T	4.5	7.3	10.2	13.0	15.9	18.7	3.8	6.0	8.1	10.3	12.5	14.6
Late	0.55	A-N	5.3	8.9	12.4	–	–	–	5.1	8.2	12.4	–	–	–
		S/T	4.7	7.6	10.5	–	–	–	4.1	6.4	8.6	–	–	–

Notes: Animal size *per se* has little effect on total requirements unless differences are extreme, but breed differences are significant. Anglo-Nubian goats have higher contents of Ca and P in milk, increasing requirement by 0.6 g Ca and 0.8 g P per kg compared with Saanen/Toggenburg. For each 10-kg difference in live weight, daily requirements will be increased or decreased by approximately 0.1 g Ca and 0.2 g P. However, if a lactating animal is gaining or losing weight, effects on Ca and P requirements may be considerable. No allowance for this has been made in Table 7.5, but live-weight gains (likely to occur in late lactation) should be allowed for by increasing daily Ca and P intakes respectively at the rate of 2.7 g and 1.6 g per 100 g daily live-weight gain. It seems unwise to reduce Ca and P intakes in anticipation of weight loss likely to occur in early lactation.

7.3.2 Requirements

Morand-Fehr and Sauvant (1978a, 1988) and Morand-Fehr *et al* (1987) concluded that there were insufficient data available to give specific recommendations on the Mg requirements of goats. Likewise, NRC (1981) provided no estimates of Mg requirements. Kessler (1984) included recommendations for Mg but did not specify the source of the basic data. The suggested availability coefficient for Mg was 0.20, with net requirements for maintenance being 3.5 mg Mg/kg live weight and 0.14 g Mg/kg milk. During the last 2 months of pregnancy, dietary allowances for Mg were suggested to be 0.5 g/d for an unspecified number of kids. The dietary allowance given for bucks was 1.5 g Mg/d, and all ages of growing female kids were suggested to need 0.5 g Mg/d.

ARC (1980) suggested that the value of 3.0 mg of Mg/kg live weight daily recommended by ARC (1965) as the faecal endogenous Mg loss for mature cattle should be adopted for cattle and sheep, and urinary excretion could be considered negligible. They also considered that, due to wide variations observed for the coefficient of absorption of Mg, an absorption coefficient of 0.294 (mean of data) should be used to calculate requirements, and a value of 0.17 used to estimate allowances, which would therefore include a safety margin. The IDWP (1984) report supported this principle.

It is suggested that until data specific to the goat are available, dietary Mg allowances should be based on the ARC (1980) recommendations for cattle and sheep (i.e. 3.0 mg of Mg/kg live weight daily). In view of the importance to goats of a regular, adequate supply of Mg, it would be appropriate to follow the principle of ARC (1980) and IDWP (1984) and adopt an absorption coefficient of 0.17 to calculate dietary allowances.

Using a value for Saanen-type goats of 0.13 g Mg/kg milk (Table 2.14), Mg requirements for milk production are 0.43 g Mg/kg milk, which is the same value as that given by ARC (1980) for Friesian cows. If goats' milk is known or believed to contain higher levels of Mg, requirements should be based on the alternative compositional data. It is suggested that the same values for Mg requirements for pregnancy according to ARC (1980) are used for the goat as for the sheep, namely 0.06 g Mg/d in the third month of pregnancy and 0.24 g Mg/d in the last 2 months, based on an assumption, but not actually specified, of an average of 1.5 foetuses. It is also suggested, that until specific data are available, Mg requirements for live-weight gain should be the 0.14 g Mg/100 g live-weight gain recommended for cattle by ARC (1980). In general, the above recommended requirements for Mg of ARC (1980) are considerably lower than those suggested by Kessler (1984), but if dietary allowances are calculated the values are relatively close.

7.4   Sodium, potassium and chloride

7.4.1   Metabolism

The metabolism of Na, K and Cl is closely inter-related (Sykes and Russel 1991) and seems similar in the goat compared to cattle and sheep (Wilke *et al* 1981; Mba 1982; Kessler 1987). Symptoms of deficiency include a depraved appetite, depressed feed intake, emaciation and reduced milk and mohair production (Haenlein 1980b, 1987).

Goats appear able to adapt to wide variations in the supply of salt (NaCl) providing that drinking water is freely available (Haenlein 1987), although Teh *et al* (1987) reported adverse effects when young does were given diets with NaCl added at 20 or 30 g/kg DM compared with 10g NaCl/kg DM. As with cattle and sheep, high K intakes by goats (e.g. 30 g K/kg DM) were found to affect Mg metabolism and retention adversely, and Na metabolism also appears to be disturbed (Kessler 1987).

The absorption efficiency for Na and K appears to be around 0.90 for goats, as for other ruminants (Kessler 1984, 1987).

7.4.2   Requirements

Requirements for K, Na and Cl by goats have not been specifically defined and it is generally assumed that recommendations for cattle and sheep may be extrapolated to goats. In practice, supplementation with Na is often required but additional K is rarely needed. The over-supply of Na is usually only of concern in specific situations, but high K intake may be a more general problem (Haenlein 1987; Kessler 1987; Sykes and Russel 1991).

NRC (1981) and Morand-Fehr (1981) suggested that diets for goats should supply 5 g NaCl/kg DM, equivalent to 2 g Na/kg diet DM, whilst Eriksson *et al* (1976) suggested 10 g NaCl/head daily plus 1.5 g NaCl/kg milk, which for most goats equates to a broadly similar dietary level. Kessler (1984) stated a net requirement for Na of 8 mg/kg live weight daily for maintenance and 0.4 g Na/kg milk, with an absorption coefficient of 0.90; under most situations this would correspond to approximately half of the dietary NaCl level suggested by NRC (1981) and Morand-Fehr (1981). Neither Eriksson *et al* (1976) nor Kessler (1984) state the basis for their recommendations.

Recommendations made by ARC (1980) and IDWP (1984) on the requirements of cattle and sheep for Na and Cl are based on very limited data. ARC (1980) suggested that sheep but not cattle may have a substantial urinary loss of Na, while IDWP (1984) considered that the pertaining experimental conditions may have created an artefact, but there were insufficient experimental data to prove this. As goats appear able to tolerate a moderate excess of Na and Cl, providing that drinking water is freely available, it is suggested that until specific data are available, the proposals of ARC (1980) for maintenance, growth and pregnancy in sheep should be adopted for the goat. Requirements for milk production by dairy animals would be more appropriately based on those for cattle.

NRC (1981) suggested for K that growing and milking goats required comparable dietary levels of K to sheep and dairy cows, namely 5 and 8 g K/kg DM respectively. Morand-Fehr *et al* (1987) and Morand-Fehr and Sauvant (1988) also suggested following guidelines for sheep and cattle; whilst Gueguen *et al* (1988) considered that K is not a problem for ruminants' nutrition and they provided no specific recommendations. Kessler (1987) assumed that, as for sheep, the minimum net endogenous requirement of goats may be 20 mg K/kg live weight and the coefficient of absorption 0.90. He also suggested a net requirement for lactation of 2.1 g K/kg milk, which implies a dietary level of about 5 g K/kg DM for a 60 kg animal giving 4 kg milk/d, with a DM intake of 3.5% of body weight.

By comparison, when Naga *et al* (1978) reduced the K intake of goats from 12 to 8 g K/kg DM, rumen microbial growth was depressed. This level of dietary K is considerably greater than that recommended by NRC (1981) or Kessler (1987), suggesting that the K requirement of goats for optimum ruminal fermentation may be greater than normal recommendations based on sheep and cattle data.

The ARC (1980) and IDWP (1984) recommendations for the K requirements of cattle and sheep were based, like those for Na and Cl, on very limited data. Furthermore, the IDWP (1984) did not accept the ARC (1980) recommendations for a number of reasons, including an apparent lack of use of an absorption coefficient for K by ARC (1980) when translating net requirements to dietary requirements. It is suggested that the higher IDWP (1984) recommendations of 5 g K/kg DM for growing sheep and 8 g K/kg DM for dairy cows should be adopted for growing kids and lactating goats respectively. Although on the basis of the report by Naga *et al* (1978) there may be benefits in higher levels of K, possible adverse effects on Mg metabolism must also be taken into account if dietary K contents are markedly greater than the above recommendations.

7.5 Copper

7.5.1 *Metabolism*

The metabolism of copper in ruminants has been extensively studied and it is well-established that complex interactions occur between Cu and a number of other elements (Underwood 1981). The metabolism of Cu and molybdenum (Mo) differs between cattle and sheep, but less is known about the metabolism of these elements in goats. Similar types of interactions almost certainly occur between Cu and other elements, but there may be quantitative differences compared to cattle and sheep (Devendra and Burns 1983; Haenlein 1980b, 1987). Søli and Nafstad (1978) and Søli and Froslie (1979) concluded that differences in Cu status between sheep and goats in Norway were difficult to explain on a nutritional basis alone.

General observations in the UK suggest that mineral supplements or feeds designed for cattle and sheep can adequately meet the Cu requirements of goats, and dairy animals can tolerate higher dietary levels of Cu than can safely be fed to sheep (Mowlem *pers comm*). There have, however, been isolated incidences of Cu toxicity when feeds containing relatively high levels of Cu and formulated for cattle have been given to goats. Humphries *et al* (1987) reported Cu poisoning in Angora doe kids imported from New Zealand, which was believed to be due to the Cu levels in the calf milk substitute used. It appeared that, like other pre-ruminant animals, the kids absorbed and accumulated Cu very efficiently, and liver Cu levels were found to be very high. The authors commented that goats develop similar symptoms of Cu toxicity to sheep, at equivalent concentrations of Cu in the liver. On the other hand, Søli and Nafstad (1978) reported that, in Norway, chronic Cu poisoning in goats appeared to be more rare than with sheep. In a toxicological experiment, although the amount of Cu administered was 3 to 4 times that which would have been used for sheep, 2 out of 3 goats had much lower liver Cu levels than would have been expected for sheep. Other workers have also found goats less susceptible than sheep to excessive Cu intakes (e.g. Ademosun and Munyabantu 1982; Economides 1986; Solaiman *et al* 1988a, b).

7.5.2   Requirements

NRC (1981) and INRA (Morand-Fehr and Sauvant 1978a; Morand-Fehr *et al* 1987; Morand-Fehr and Sauvant 1988) considered that guidelines for cattle and sheep requirements should be followed for goats, taking into account dietary Mo levels. Lamand (1981) suggested a deficiency limit minimum of 7 mg Cu/kg DM for goats, but at dietary Mo concentrations above 3 mg Mo/kg DM, dietary S levels and possibly zinc (Zn) and manganese (Mn) concentrations should be taken into account. Ademosun and Munyabantu (1982) found that giving West African dwarf goats a Cu supplement to increase total dietary Cu levels to around 8 to 10 mg Cu/kg DM improved kid growth rates. Gueguen *et al* (1988) suggested that ruminant diets should contain a minimum of 7 mg Cu/kg DM but preferably 10 mg Cu/kg DM, and that diets containing over 3 mg Mo/kg DM should be avoided.

It is suggested that the ARC (1980) factorial approach to the calculation of Cu requirements should be adopted for goats. This approach was supported by IDWP (1984) for cattle and sheep, and provided further information to adjust for the effects of dietary antagonists, particularly S and Mo. The recommended level of Cu for cattle, calculated to be about 12 mg Cu/kg DM under normal conditions, should adequately supply the needs of goats, but from the previously quoted evidence the calculated normal recommendation for sheep of about 6 mg Cu/kg DM may be too low. A guideline recommendation for Cu requirements is given in Table 7.6.

Table 7.6: Summary of trace element requirements for goats.

Element	Suggested requirement (mg/kg diet DM)
Copper	10 to 20
Zinc	50 to 80
Cobalt	0.11 to 0.20
Iodine	0.15 to 2.0
Manganese	60 to 120
Iron	30 to 40
Selenium	0.05

7.5.3 Toxicity

Sheep are more susceptible to Cu toxicity than cattle, although the actual threshold value for dietary Cu varies with factors such as presence of dietary antagonists and length of time of feeding (ARC 1980). It appears that while goats may be less susceptible to Cu toxicity than sheep, they may be less tolerant than cattle (NRC 1981; Morand-Fehr and Sauvant 1978a, 1988). In their recommendations for goats, Morand-Fehr *et al* (1987) did not make a clear statement on dietary Cu levels likely to result in toxicity. Lamand (1981) suggested an upper toxicity limit of 30 mg Cu/kg DM, whilst Gueguen *et al* (1988) suggested that the upper limit for goat diets was 20 mg Cu/kg DM, compared with 15 and 30 mg Cu/kg DM for sheep and cattle diets respectively. Virtually nothing is known about differences between breeds, nor between fibre-producing and dairy goats, but Humphries *et al* (1987) suggested that Angoras may be more susceptible to Cu toxicity than other breeds. Furthermore, pre-ruminant and growing lambs appear to absorb Cu more efficiently than do calves, and Humphries *et al* (1987) suggested that young kids may be more similar to lambs than calves in this respect.

In view of the lack of knowledge for goats, and particularly fibre-producing goats, it would be prudent to follow toxicity guidelines given by ARC (1980) and IDWP (1984) for sheep, and to take into account the INRA recommendation of a maximum dietary Cu level of 20 mg Cu/kg DM (Gueguen *et al* 1988).

7.6   Requirements for other trace elements

Information on the requirements by goats for other trace elements is extremely sparse. There are few experimental or observational data to contradict the assumption that goats require broadly similar amounts of the same trace elements as other ruminants, and in general deficiency symptoms in goats appear to be similar to those in cattle and sheep. The relatively low incidence of some mineral deficiencies in goats may be due either to differences in requirements or to differences in diet composition and level of production (Haenlein 1980b, 1987; NRC 1981; Morand-Fehr and Sauvant 1978a, 1988; Morand-Fehr *et al* 1987).

The adoption of trace element requirements recommended for cattle and sheep as suitable for goats is complicated by the fact that in many instances the requirements of cattle and sheep are not clearly established. It is also well-known that many interactions occur between different inorganic elements in the diet, which may influence requirements, but these have generally not been clarified or quantitatively defined.

In this section trace element requirements of cattle and sheep proposed by ARC (1980) and IDWP (1984) are reviewed, and the recommended dietary concentrations for goats, summarised in Table 7.6, are discussed in the light of the sparse data specific to goats. In general, it is proposed that recommendations for dairy cattle should be adopted for dairy goats, and requirements for fibre goats and growing kids considered to be similar to those for sheep.

7.6.1   Zinc

ARC (1980), from a factorial approach, concluded that 30 mg Zn/kg dietary DM should meet requirements fully. IDWP (1984) considered that this value was minimal, particularly in view of dietary interactions and between-animal variations, and it suggested an allowance of 40 mg Zn/kg DM. Lamand (1981), on the basis of the French goat research programme, suggested 45 mg Zn/kg DM under normal circumstances but 75 mg Zn/kg DM in the presence of interacting elements.

In practice, up to 150 mg Zn/kg DM appears to be well-tolerated by ruminants (ARC 1980), and even higher levels often do not have observable adverse effects. Taking this into account, together with evidence that development of the reproductive organs requires relatively high Zn intakes (Chhabra and Arora 1985) and the possible presence of interacting dietary components, it seems prudent to consider that Zn requirements for goats are higher than those suggested by ARC (1980) for cattle and sheep. Until more specific data are available, it is suggested that diets for goats should contain at least 50 mg Zn/kg DM, and possibly up to 80 mg Zn/kg DM for breeding females or in the presence of dietary Zn antagonists.

7.6.2 Cobalt

ARC (1980) and IDWP (1984) suggested that a cobalt (Co) level in cattle and sheep diets of 0.11 mg Co/kg DM should usually meet Co requirements, although high-concentrate diets should contain 0.2 mg Co/kg DM. Lamand (1981) considered that goats require 0.1 mg Co/kg DM, and it is therefore suggested that the ARC (1980) recommendation of 0.11 mg Co/kg DM should be adopted for goats. It also seems prudent to increase dietary levels to 0.2 mg Co/kg DM for high-concentrate diets.

In general the toxicity of Co is low, but cattle may be less tolerant of high intakes than sheep (ARC 1980). The situation with goats is unknown and, as suggested by ARC (1980) for other ruminants, rations for goats should not exceed 30 mg Co/kg DM. It may even be advisable to follow the recommendation of Gueguen *et al* (1988) that ruminant rations should contain no more than 10 mg Co/kg DM.

7.6.3 Iodine

In the absence of goitrogens, ARC (1980) recommended that a dietary iodine (I) level of 0.5 mg I/kg DM should be adequate for pregnant and lactating cattle and sheep. In summer requirements might be lower, perhaps 0.15 mg I/kg DM, but in the presence of goitrogens dietary concentrations should be increased to 2 mg I/kg DM. IDWP (1984) accepted these recommendations, and it is suggested that the same values are adopted for goats. Gueguen *et al* (1988) recommended values for ruminants similar to those of ARC (1980) and the values given by Lamand (1981) from experience with goats, also support the current proposal.

ARC (1980) suggested a maximum safe dietary level of 8 to 20 mg I/kg DM for cattle and sheep, which should also be adopted for goats.

7.6.4 Manganese

Manganese (Mn) requirements have not been clearly established for any ruminant species, and it seems likely that they will vary considerably according to dietary interactions. ARC (1980) suggested a dietary concentration of 20 to 25 mg Mn/kg DM but IDWP (1984) considered this to be minimal and proposed a dietary level of 40 mg Mn/kg DM. Lamand (1981) suggested diets for goats should contain 60 mg Mn/kg DM, with up to 120 mg Mn/kg DM in the presence of interacting factors, but in contrast, Haenlein (1987) proposed that goats may require about 20 mg Mn/kg diet.

In view of the disparity in recommended values, the lack of data specific to goats, and the reasonable margin between dietary requirements and levels which cause problems of toxicity or interference with other elements, it is suggested that the Mn requirement of goats should be taken as the relatively high value of 60 mg Mn/kg DM proposed by Lamand (1981). If in some situations Mn is over-supplied, this is likely to be of little consequence and the risk of a deficiency developing should be low.

7.6.5 *Iron*

Lamand (1981) suggested that goat diets should have an iron (Fe) content of at least 30 mg Fe/kg DM, but Guegen *et al* (1988) considered that low Fe supplies for ruminants should not be a problem, except possibly for milk-fed animals. However, Haenlein (1987) suggested that the Fe supply of newborn kids may be more critical than that for calves and lambs and, as internal parasites were more often a serious problem in goats, higher Fe supplements might be needed than for cattle.

In practice, goats kept under good management systems in temperate countries should have a low parasite burden, and it is suggested that the dietary requirements of 30 to 40 mg Fe/kg DM proposed by ARC (1980) and IDWP (1984) for cattle and sheep should be adequate for goats. As with other ruminants, excessive intakes of Fe should be avoided to reduce the risk of interference in the metabolism of other inorganic elements.

7.6.6 *Selenium and vitamin E*

Although selenium (Se)/vitamin E deficiencies have rarely been reported (Haenlein 1980b, 1987; Devendra and Burns 1983) goats require both Se and vitamin E (Volker and Steinberg 1981; Kessler *et al* 1986). ARC (1980) suggested that dietary levels of 0.03 to 0.05 mg Se/kg DM are marginal for cattle and sheep and, as a provisional guide, growing or pregnant sheep and cattle required a minimum of 10 to 15 mg vitamin E/kg DM; higher levels may be needed if Se intakes are low or marginal. IDWP (1984) stressed that these recommendations should be regarded as minimal.

The ARC (1980) and IDWP (1984) recommendations are in line with those suggested by Lamand (1981) and Gueguen *et al* (1988), and it is therefore proposed that they should be adopted for goats, at least until more specific data are available. As with cattle and sheep, precise dietary requirements will be influenced by the relative levels of Se or vitamin E in the diet, and the presence of unsaturated fats.

Se is a relatively toxic element and the tolerance level of 3 mg Se/kg diet DM suggested by ARC (1980) for ruminants should be regarded as a maximum value, unless proven otherwise for goats.

7.7   Requirements for vitamins

Published data on the vitamin requirements of goats, reviewed by Volker and Steinberg (1981), and Haenlein (1987), are extremely sparse. There appears to be no information available on the effects of vitamins on the production and composition of goats' milk, and on its vitamin content (Morand-Fehr and Sauvant 1980). Morand-Fehr and Sauvant (1978a, 1988), Morand-Fehr *et al* (1987) and Kessler (1984) made only a general reference to the need to ensure that rations supply adequate vitamins, particularly the fat-soluble vitamins A, D_3 and E, and Morand-Fehr and Sauvant (1988) referred to requirements based on other ruminants given by Wolter (1988). The recommendations for vitamin A and vitamin D given by NRC (1981) for goats of different live weights and levels and types of production were extrapolated from those recommended for cattle and sheep.

The apparently low incidence of observed vitamin deficiencies may arise because in many areas goats are not kept intensively, they have a relatively low level of production and their choice of feeds is wide. Goats with a fully developed rumen can synthesise adequate amounts of the vitamin B complex, vitamin C and vitamin K, but they require dietary sources of vitamins A, D_3 and E. Young kids require the vitamin B complex in the diet until their rumen develops.

Volker and Steinberg (1981) concluded that it was probably more satisfactory to extrapolate the requirements of goats for vitamins from those suggested for cattle and sheep, than to summarise the results of feeding trials with goats. It is therefore suggested that, in view of the wide range of values for recommended requirements quoted in the literature and the lack of data specific to goats, the vitamin requirements of goats are considered to be similar to those of cattle and sheep, as summarised by ARC (1980) and IDWP (1984).

8.   Production

8.1   Rearing kids to weaning

8.1.1   Introduction

Like all aspects of goat production, when discussing rearing and research that has been carried out to investigate rearing strategies it must be recognised that goats throughout the world are kept in widely different systems and environments. This brings into question the value of considering or comparing some work in tropical or developing countries with that in more sophisticated "western" environments. The majority of goats in the world are in very different environments and are largely of very different breed types from those found in Europe, the USA and Australasia.

8.1.2   Systems

A variety of rearing systems is used for goats including natural rearing, particularly with fibre-producing breeds, artificial rearing of herd replacements and various systems for meat kids. Naturally reared kids are normally left with their dams until about 1 month before the start of the normal breeding season, which generally means the kids are 12 to 16 weeks of age.

(a)   Dairy goat kids

Where milk is required for sale or for other reasons, kids are artificially reared from birth or soon after. A variety of regimes can be used, as Mowlem (1988) has recorded (see Table 8.1). A number of milk substitutes are available, some produced specifically for kids, some for calves and some for lambs (Mowlem 1984). These mainly comprise skim-milk powder with added fat, although some contain whey powder with added soya protein. In general, crude protein levels are within the range 220 to 360 g/kg and the fat content varies from 120 to 260 g/kg. Some milk substitutes, particularly those formulated for calves, contain growth promoters such as virginiamycin. The recommended concen-

Table 8.1: Examples of artificial kid rearing regimes (Mowlem 1988).

Early weaning at 6 or 8 weeks[1]		Weaning at 10 weeks		
Age (weeks)	Milk offered	Age (weeks)	Number of feeds per day	Quantity per feed (ml)
4(6)	*Ad libitum*	1–6	3	750
5(7)	Half amount consumed last day of week 4(6)	7–8	2	850
6(8)	Half amount consumed last day of week 5(7)	9	2	570
7(9)	No milk	11	no milk	–

[1] Figures in brackets refer to 8-week weaning.

tration of milk powder in the liquid also varies from 125 to 200 g/kg for different products, and the recommended feeding temperature from ambient to 42°C.

The presentation of the milk feed may be by open bucket or trough, a lamb-bar type of teat feeder or an automatic milk feeding machine. Some workers have suggested that trough or bucket feeding leads to problems, with kids drinking too quickly and with milk entering the rumen and causing bloat. A system was used for many years at the former National Institute for Research in Dairying, where all kids (about 100 per year) were reared by feeding them warm goats' milk in open troughs (Mowlem 1972). No problems with bloat were observed.

In a working situation some farmers have experienced problems rearing kids on automatic machines. It appears that unknown factors may trigger off excessive drinking, which in turn causes diarrhoea. This results in dehydration, and more drinking. Usually kids seem to recover from this situation themselves, and once they reach 3 to 4 weeks of age they seem able to cope with this sort of challenge.

When milk substitutes are offered *ad libitum*, it is difficult to feed them except in some form of feeder where the milk is dispensed via teats. Kids clamber over everything possible and open troughs or buckets are quickly fouled. It is only possible to use troughs and buckets if kids are given a limited amount and if they are supervised while drinking. There are a number of lamb-bar type teat feeder designs and most are satisfactory, although those with teats fixed directly into the milk container seem to give the best results. It is important that milk feeders for kids are fitted with lids otherwise the feed soon becomes fouled by active kids dangling their feet into the milk.

Milk substitutes are formulated for feeding warm or at ambient temperatures. Most reports agree that ambient temperatures are preferable. Warming is only suitable for rationed feeds. With *ad libitum* systems kids tend to drink warm feeds to excess and also the feeds do not remain warm for long. This means that over the period between feeder replenishments the kids drink milk of varying temperature, which may contribute to scouring problems.

For all rearing regimes the kids should be encouraged to eat solid food, such as calf or lamb rearing concentrates and good hay, from 2 to 3 weeks of age. It is important that they are encouraged to drink water at this time and a clean supply should always be available.

(b) Fibre-producing goat kids

Most cashmere and Angora kids are naturally reared in management systems akin to those pertaining in sheep flocks. Weaning normally takes place at about 14 weeks of age, although entire male kids are generally weaned at no later than 12 weeks old, by which age they can be sexually mature.

Performance, measured in terms of growth rate, is thus largely dependent on the intake of nutrients from milk, particularly in the first few weeks, and on the intake of solid food, which will generally be herbage, supplemented in some cases with creep feed.

The composition of goats' milk varies markedly between breeds and with stage of lactation; consequently, early kid growth rate is more closely related to the intake of nutrients, particularly energy, from milk than to milk yield *per se*. Russel and Adkins (1990) found that milk fat content was negatively related to milk yield (r = −0.65) and positively to protein content (r = 0.55).

In cashmere goat kids, born following embryo transfer and reared by their feral, feral × dairy, and dairy breed surrogate dams, Russel and Adkins (1990) observed significant relationships between kid performance and estimated milk fat intake over weeks 3 to 10 of lactation in the feral and dairy breed groups (see Table 8.2). The relationships were:

Feral $\quad\quad \triangle W$ (g/d) = 0.797 ($\pm$ 0.251) FI + 97.0 (r = 0.71; p < 0.05)
Feral × dairy $\triangle W$ (g/d) = 0.930 ($\pm$ 0.543) FI + 89.3 (r = 0.42; NS)
Dairy $\quad\quad \triangle W$ (g/d) = 0.815 ($\pm$ 0.370) FI + 86.0 (r = 0.57; p < 0.05)
where $\quad\quad \triangle W \quad$ = daily live-weight gain (g) and FI = daily milk fat intake (g).

There is little information available on the nutrient intakes needed to support the levels of milk production required for satisfactory kid growth rates. Most fibre-producing goats rear their kids while grazing and the present evidence suggests that on sown pastures sward height should be maintained in the 7- to 9-cm range to ensure high levels of voluntary feed intake. In the early part of the season, before sward heights have attained this level, supplementary concentrates containing a source of low degradability protein should be provided.

Table 8.2: Milk production and composition, and performance of cashmere kids reared on different dam genotypes (data refer to weeks 3 to 10 of lactation; Russel and Adkins 1990).

Genotype of dam	Feral	Feral × dairy	Dairy
Number of kids reared	1	1	2
Mean milk production (kg/d)	1.27±0.41	1.90±0.26	2.99±0.67
Mean fat content (g/kg)	70	49	31
Mean protein content (g/kg)	34	35	26
Mean fat production (g/d)	85.6±22.8	92.2±14.3	91.4±22.1
Mean protein production (g/d)	43.5±13.2	65.3±10.5	77.9±16.3
Mean kid growth rate (g/d)	165±25.2	175±25.7	161±29.4

8.1.3   Responses and requirements

(a)   Voluntary dry matter intake

Published data on voluntary DM intakes in kids are scarce, they are expressed in many different ways and they vary considerably, partly due to breed differences. It would seem that more work is needed in this area.

Havrevoll *et al* (1985) recorded an average daily intake of 432 g DM in kids from birth to 10 weeks of age, during which time the average daily gain was 142 g. Morand-Fehr *et al*, (1982) recorded a DM intake of 214 g/d, or 29.2 g/kg $W^{0.75}$ daily, for Alpine kids at 6 weeks of age.

Abrams *et al* (1985) investigated the DM intake of milk-fed Anglo-Nubian kids fed whole milk or milk substitute of two different concentrations, with unexpected results. The whole milk group had an average DM intake of 90 g/d from birth to 6 weeks, which produced an average daily gain of 93 g. The group fed the high-concentration milk substitute (180 g DM/kg) had an average DM intake of 124 g/d, producing an average daily gain of 73 g, but with the lower concentration milk substitute (135 g DM/kg), DM intake was only 71 g/d and average daily gain only 19 g.

(b)   Energy

Morand-Fehr *et al* (1982) cited a number of reports giving the daily metabolisable energy requirements for maintenance and growth recorded from experimental work with a variety of breeds (Table 8.3).

Morand-Fehr and Sauvant (1978a) recommended, for kids up to 30 days of age and averaging 6.5 kg live weight and a daily gain of 165 g, an allowance of 782 kJ NE/kg $W^{0.75}$ daily. For kids between 30 and 60 days, averaging 11.5 kg live weight and with the same average daily gain of 165 g, the recommendation was 577 kJ NE/kg $W^{0.75}$ daily.

Morand-Fehr *et al* (1987) recommended energy values for live-weight gain (EV_g) of 10.04 MJ/kg gain for kids of 1 month of age and 14.6 MJ/kg gain for kids of 7 months of age.

Table 8.3: Estimates of energy requirements for growth.

Breed	Daily ME allowance (kJ/g weight gain)	Reference
Kambing Katjang	45.2	Devendra (1967)
Norwegian	26.0	Opstvedt (1967)
West African Dwarf	21.5	Akinsoyinu (1974)
"Indian"	26.9	Rajpoot *et al* (1979)

(c)   Protein

Data on protein requirements or responses are even more scarce. Morand-Fehr *et al* (1982) recommended 19.7 g DCP/kg $W^{0.75}$ daily for kids up to 30 days of age averaging 6.5 kg live weight, and 12.7 g DCP/kg $W^{0.75}$ daily for kids between 30 and 60 days and averaging 11.5 kg live weight.

8.1.4   Practical feeding

The conclusion of Mowlem (1984) and Morand-Fehr (*pers comm*) was that, if kids are weaned early (i.e. 5 to 6 weeks of age) the type of milk substitute is not important. Both workers agreed that kids do not grow well on grass, probably because of parasite challenges and energy losses due to exercise. Morand-Fehr *et al* (1982) recommended weaning at 5 weeks if health and feed intakes were good, and they suggested a minimum intake of milk powder of 40 g DM/kg $W^{0.75}$ daily with 30 to 40 g/d of solid feed. Most workers agree that weight rather than age is a better parameter for weaning, and Owen and de Paiva (1980) concluded that kids could be weaned as early as 4 weeks without major problems.

Various workers have investigated milk substitute concentrations and there is some variance in opinion about the optimum. A range of 140 to 260 g/kg has been reported. Morand-Fehr *et al* (1982) suggested that 240 g/kg is the maximum that kids can tolerate. Mowlem (1979) investigated the performance of kids fed milk substitute (240 g CP and 140 g fat/kg) at 100, 140 and 175 g/kg and concluded that 100 g/kg was too low and 175 g/kg did not give an economic improvement compared to 140 g/kg. Most workers agree that it is preferable to offer milk substitutes at ambient temperature.

Morand-Fehr *et al* (1982) reported that soya protein reduced digestibility. Tanabe and Kameoka (1977) showed that substitution of soya for milk protein caused a reduction in digestibility, with a consequent reduction in weight gain, but Mowlem (1985) found that milk feeds comprising alcohol-treated soya protein and whey gave satisfactory growth rates when compared with feeds incorporating skim milk.

Nitzan *et al* (1985) reported satisfactory weight gains from kids fed milk substitute with an added starch and soya protein mix. Week-old kids gained weight at 232 g/d to a live weight of 19.6 kg when given the normal milk substitute, and 226 g/d when given milk substitute containing 300 g/kg of the soya protein mix.

Pre-weaning growth rate is influenced by breed type as well as nutrition, with a range of 90 to 240 g/d having been reported. Russel and Adkins (1990) recorded a smaller daily weight gain in feral kids than feral × dairy kids (Table 8.2). Although the milk from the feral does had a higher fat content, differences in yield, giving different total fat intakes, would explain the different kid performances. Presumably the daily gain from dairy kids (161±29.4 g/d) was least because the increased milk yield did not compensate for reduced milk quality, and these does were also feeding, on average, twin kids.

8.2 Nutrition of the dairy goat

8.2.1 Rearing

In normal commercial production, the aim is to mate kids at 7 months of age to kid at 12 months. To achieve this the weight of the kids at mating should be at least 60% of adult weight, i.e. 40 to 45 kg for Saanen-type goats, which requires a relatively high pre-mating live-weight gain of about 150 g/d (Wilkinson and Stark 1987a). Feeding after mating must allow for continued growth as well as for development of the foetus. It is preferable that these aims are achieved mainly by the use of high-quality forages rather than by excessive reliance on starchy concentrates, which can cause over-fattening.

8.2.2 Pregnancy

As with the dairy cow, nutrition in the last third of pregnancy in the goat has important influences on subsequent lactational performance. Goats should kid with adequate fat reserves to sustain high yields in the early stages of lactation. However over-feeding concentrates in late pregnancy probably gives little or no benefit in subsequent milk production and may even be detrimental (Morand-Fehr and Sauvant 1978b). Moreover, forage intake in lactation appears to be stimulated by high forage intake in late pregnancy (Morand-Fehr and Sauvant 1978b; Oldham *et al* 1983), so high-concentrate feeding before parturition could also be detrimental in that respect.

Morand-Fehr and Sauvant (1978b) recommended that a suitable feeding regime in the last third of pregnancy should therefore be based on high-quality forages available *ad libitum* with concentrates increasing to about 0.5 kg/d by parturition, though Skjevdal (1981) recommended that this should be varied from 0.1 to 0.8 kg/d, depending on the age and yield potential of the goat.

Ketosis sometimes occurs in late pregnancy in goats carrying multiple foetuses and should be treated as for other ruminants.

8.2.3   Milk production

After parturition milk yield increases rapidly to a peak and then declines slowly. Goats are normally dried off after about 10 months of lactation, in preparation for kidding at 12-month intervals. Dairy goats have the ability to continue milking for a second year, though at a lower level than in the first year, without being mated a second time. However, this does not form part of normal commercial practice.

Peak milk yield occurs about 6 to 8 weeks after parturition in most breeds (Knowles and Watkin 1938; Lu *et al* 1984; Badamana *et al* 1990) and was found to be one week later in primiparous compared to multiparous Alpine goats (Randy *et al* 1988). According to Knowles and Watkin (1938), milk yield remains fairly constant for about 3 months before declining, the rate of decline being slower in British Saanens than in other, lower-yielding breeds (including Anglo-Nubians, British Alpines and Toggenburgs). However, in more recent studies with British Saanens, peak milk yield was maintained for only 1 to 2 weeks (Badamana *et al* 1990). The rate of decline in milk yield has not been widely reported but was found to be proportionately 0.035 and 0.028 per week in Alpine goats given 0.64 or 1.21 kg concentrates daily in mid-lactation (Morand-Fehr and Sauvant 1980). Recently, however, the lactation curves of white British dairy goats have been studied by Williams (1993a, b). An empirical model for the lactation curve was developed and the effects of farm, parity, season and litter studied. He derived an equation :

$$Y \ (kg/d) = A*exp\{-0.618(1 + (t1)/2)*t1 - 0.0707(t1)^2 - 1.01/t\}$$

where t is the day of lactation, $t1 = (t - 150)/100$ and $A = 2.65 \pm 0.82$.

Typical predicted average and above average milk yields (+1 standard deviation) at various stages of the lactation are given in Table 8.4.

Table 8.4: Predicted daily milk yields (kg/d) of dairy goats by stage of lactation, according to Williams (1993a, b)[1].

	Week of lactation										
	2	6	10	14	18	22	26	30	34	38	42
Above average[2]	4.8	5.0	4.8	4.4	3.9	3.4	2.8	2.2	1.7	1.2	0.9
Average	3.7	3.8	3.7	3.4	3.0	2.6	2.1	1.7	1.3	0.9	0.7

[1] Calculated with A = 2.65 (see Section 8.2.3).
[2] Calculated with A = 3.47, i.e. one standard deviation (0.82) added.

8.2.4   Live-weight change during lactation

In Section 2.1.4, it was noted that the extent of live-weight changes in lactating goats varies considerably, but that mobilisation of body fat and protein reserves undoubtedly occurs. INRA (1988) suggested that goats lose about 1 kg adipose tissue/week for the first month post-partum and 0.5 kg/week for a further month. From about the fourth month of lactation, dairy goats begin to regain live weight. INRA (1988) recommended a target of 1.2 kg live-weight gain/month for multiparous goats and 2.2 kg/month for primiparous. The INRA estimates of live-weight change are accepted and used in the calculation of energy and protein requirements of lactating goats.

The composition of both live-weight losses and gains and the energy and protein contribution to milk production or requirements for gain were discussed earlier in Section 2.1.4. The Working Party agreed to adopt the ARC (1980) [EV_g] value of 23.9 MJ/kg live-weight change as appropriate for nominal live-weight losses and gains in lactating goats. For net protein value [NP_g], the ARC (1980) recommendation for the composition of live-weight loss in lactating cattle and sheep of 138 g NP_g/kg live-weight is adopted here.

8.2.5   Voluntary feed intake

Voluntary feed intake increases steadily after parturition and usually reaches a peak during the third month of lactation, though this varies considerably (Lu *et al* 1984; Randy *et al* 1988; Badamana *et al* 1990). Since peak feed intake normally occurs later than peak milk yield, as in dairy cows, it is important that the feed offered during this period should be of high quality, though not too rich in concentrates (Morand-Fehr and Sauvant 1978b; Skjevdal 1981). Published estimates of DM intake by lactating goats were reviewed in Section 4 and Table 4.3.

8.2.6   Milk yield responses

Milk yield is highly correlated with ME intake, the correlation increasing as lactation progresses (Morand-Fehr and Sauvant 1978b; Skjevdal 1981). Morand-Fehr and Sauvant (1978b) suggested that the energy quality of the diet was better described in terms of its ME concentration (q_m or M/D) rather than forage:concentrate ratio and that maximum yield was obtained with diets with M/D values of 9.4 to 10.0 MJ ME/kg DM in the third and fifth month of lactation and 8.8 to 9.4 MJ ME/kg DM in the seventh month. Higher or lower ME concentrations caused milk yield to fall. This response pattern conflicts with observations with dairy cows, where milk yield would be expected to increase with increases in the ME concentration of the diet to at least 12.0 MJ/kg DM.

Milk yield response to extra concentrates by dairy cows with free access to forage varies widely and is greatly influenced by the substitution rate (decrease in forage DM intake per unit increase in concentrate DM intake), which itself is highly variable. From a review of French and Norwegian literature, Skjevdal (1981) found that substitution rate in dairy goats varied from 0.2 to 0.8 but with most values around 0.5 to 0.6. Results of experiments with British Saanen goats are in agreement with this (Oldham *et al* 1984). In view of this wide variation in substitution rates, it is not surprising that the milk yield responses to extra concentrates in goats consuming various forages *ad libitum* in reports from Norway, France and the UK vary from about 0.4 to 1.6 kg milk/kg concentrate DM (Morand-Fehr and Sauvant 1980; Skjevdal 1981; Oldham *et al* 1985).

Increasing dietary CP concentration to at least 180 to 200 g/kg DM is reflected in increased feed intake and milk yield in dairy cows. With British Saanen goats in early to mid lactation, intake of hay (86 to 109 g CP/kg DM) increased when the CP in the concentrates was increased to about 180 g/kg DM (about 130 to 140 g CP/kg diet DM) but it did not respond to higher CP concentrations (Badamana and Sutton 1987; Badamana *et al* 1990). Results of some experiments have indicated little benefit in milk yield to increasing dietary CP concentrations above about 150 g/kg DM (Lindahl 1955, 1956; Lu *et al* 1984; Badamana and Sutton 1987; Badamana *et al* 1990) but others have shown responses to increases up to about 180 to 200 g CP/kg diet DM (Ciszuk 1980; Skjevdal 1981; Ciszuk and Lindberg 1988). The importance of the N source in determining responses was apparent from the work of Ciszuk and Lindberg (1988), who found a response to CP concentrations up to about 200 g/kg diet DM with fishmeal but not with urea as the N supplement to a basal diet containing about 130g CP/kg DM. This difference they calculated to reflect the supply of truly absorbed AA-N to the duodenum, with a curvilinear response of milk N plus maintenance N to the concentration of truly absorbed amino acids in the feed OM. Skjevdal (1981) also showed a greater milk yield response to fishmeal than to soyabean meal.

8.2.7   Metabolic diseases

Metabolic diseases are not generally a serious problem in goats, but ketosis can occur during both pregnancy and early lactation, whilst hypocalcaemia and hypomagnesaemia can affect lactating goats. The risk of hypomagnesaemia can be averted by supplying a Mg supplement when goats are turned out to pasture. Urolithiasis can also affect intensively fed male goats.

1)   Ketosis

Sauvant *et al* (1991) reviewed the mechanism and factors affecting the incidence of ketosis in pregnant and lactating goats. The disorder is the result of a discrepancy between glucose demand for the foetuses or for milk production, and glucose availability from the diet, resulting in body lipid mobilisation to increase glucose supply. Incomplete metabolism of mobilised body fat in the liver results in the accumulation of ketone bodies in the blood, causing the symptoms of toxicity observed. The primary cause is a deficit in energy intake, as with cattle and sheep. Sauvant *et al* (1991) state that the incidence of ketosis is higher in pregnant than lactating goats, possibly because the lactating goat can reduce glucose demand by reducing milk yield. The link between diet energy density and voluntary feed intake and level of animal productivity is also quite clear. Several animal factors interact to affect the level of blood ketones; body fatness, stage of pregnancy, number of kids carried and milk yield, with late pregnancy and early lactation being the main risk periods. The treatment of ketosis has been described by Guss (1977). Prevention of ketosis is normally a matter of reformulating the diet to increase daily energy intake, usually by increasing the proportion of concentrates in the diet. High dietary protein levels may increase the incidence with goats in good body condition, as it increases the rate of fat mobilisation, raising blood ketone body levels.

2)   Hypocalcaemia

Hypocalcaemia, or "milk fever", has been reported in dairy goats (Haenlein 1987) but the evidence from general observation (Haenlein 1984; Mowlem *pers comm*) is that goats are less susceptible to this disorder than cattle at comparable levels of production. This may be due to hormone responses during the period of high Ca demand following lactation, to differences in typical diets fed to goats compared with dairy cows, or to differences in type and/or level of stress imposed at or near parturition. Both Ca intake and Ca/P ratio should be controlled in late pregnancy to reduce this risk.

3)   Urolithiasis

Male kids are highly susceptible to this disease if they are fed on high cereal diets, requiring the addition of buffers to avoid them going off feed with acidosis. If alkaline urine results, then crystals of magnesium ammonium phosphate are precipitated, blocking the urethra. As with intensively fed lambs, the addition of Ca to maintain a Ca/P ratio of 2:1 in the diet and the avoidance of the addition of any Mg compounds is effective in preventing the occurrence of this disorder.

8.2.8   Requirements and feed intake capacity

Examples of daily requirements for ME and MP for goats at different stages of lactation, based on earlier chapters, are set out in Tables 8.5 and 8.6. They are based on a 65-kg British Saanen/Toggenburg goat consuming a diet with a q_m value of 0.6, M/D = 11.3 MJ ME/kg DM. These requirements must be met within the intake capacity of the goat, as discussed earlier, and these limits, as defined in INRA (1988), are set out in Table 8.7. Reservations about

Table 8.5: Estimates of the requirements for metabolisable energy (MJ/d) for multiparous British Saanen/Toggenburg goats throughout the lactation cycle, assuming a mean live weight of 65 kg and a value of 0.6 for q_m (ME/GE)[1].

Milk yield (kg/d)	Month of lactation				Dry and pregnant	
	1[2]	2–3	4–9[3]	10[3,4]	11[3,4]	12[3,4]
0	–	–	13.0	15.1	17.7	20.6
1	11.7	16.4	17.6	19.7	–	–
2	16.3	21.1	22.3	24.3	–	–
3	21.0	25.8	27.0	29.1	–	–
4	25.7	30.6	31.8	–	–	–
5	30.5	35.5	36.7	–	–	–
6	35.4	40.4	41.6	–	–	–

[1] Increase requirements by approximately 0.8 MJ ME/kg milk for Anglo-Nubians.
[2] Assuming live-weight loss of 1 kg/week, reducing requirements at maintenance by 4.6 MJ ME/d.
[3] Assuming live-weight gain of 1.2 kg/month, requiring 1.5 MJ ME/d. For primiparous goats, a further 3.9 MJ ME/d for growth should be added.
[4] Months 10, 11 and 12 are equivalent to months 3, 4 and 5 of pregnancy, and estimates assume 2 foetuses; for 3 foetuses, a further 0.5, 1.4 and 2.1 MJ ME/d for months 10, 11, and 12 respectively should be added.

Table 8.6: Estimates of the requirements for metabolisable protein (MP), (g/d) for multiparous 65-kg Saanen/Toggenburg goats[1] throughout the lactation cycle.

Milk yield (kg/d)	Month of lactation			Drying off and pregnant[3,4]		
	1[2]	2–3	4–9[3]	10(3)	11(4)	12(5)
0	–	–	57	71	80	95
1	61	91	96	109	–	–
2	99	129	133	147	–	–
3	138	168	172	186	–	–
4	176	206	210	–	–	–
5	215	245	249	–	–	–
6	253	283	287	–	–	–

[1] Increase requirements by 9 g MP/kg milk for Anglo-Nubians.
[2] A deficit of 30 g/d MP is accepted in month 1 of lactation.
[3] Assuming life-weight gain of 1.2 kg/month, equivalent to 4 g MP/d. For primiparous goats, a further 9 g MP/d should be added to allow a growth rate of 2.2 kg/month.
[4] Months 10, 11 and 12 are equivalent to months 3, 4 and 5 of pregnancy respectively. Estimates assume 2 foetuses; for 3 foetuses a further 3.8, 7.8, and 11.0 g/d of MP for months 10, 11 and 12 respectively should be added (see Table 6.6).

Table 8.7: Estimates of maximum intakes of dry matter (DM, kg/d) of dairy goats at various stages of lactation, assuming diets based on maize silage, lucerne hay and concentrates, and a mean live weight of 65 kg (INRA 1988).

Milk yield (kg/d)	Weeks of lactation				Month of lactation			
	1	2	3	4	2 – dry	8–10[1]	11[1]	12[1]
0	–	–	–	–	1.40	1.40	1.40	1.28
1	1.23	1.42	1.54	1.62	1.71	–	–	–
2	1.45	1.67	1.82	1.91	2.01	–	–	–
3	1.67	1.93	2.11	2.20	2.32	–	–	–
4	1.89	2.17	2.36	2.49	2.62	–	–	–
5	2.11	2.43	2.64	2.78	2.93	–	–	–
6	–	2.68	2.91	3.07	3.23	–	–	–

[1] Equivalent to months 1 to 3, 4 and 5 of pregnancy respectively.

the basis of these estimates of the intake capacity of goats were discussed earlier.

8.3   Nutrition of fibre goats

8.3.1   Mohair from Angora goats

Australian work indicates that mohair production is sensitive to level of nutrition (McGregor 1984, 1986). Angora goats grazed at a low stocking rate (7.5/ha) grew more mohair than those at a high stocking rate (12.5/ha). The implied difference in nutrient intake also affected fibre quality in two respects. Firstly, the higher level of nutrition (low stocking rate) adversely affected mean fibre diameter, which increased from 24.1 to 28.0 μm and from 27.9 to 32.3 μm in 2- and 3.5-year-old animals respectively. Regression analysis showed that mean fibre diameter increased by 0.26 (±0.04) μm per kg increase in live weight. In animals fed in individual pens, the increase in fibre diameter per kg increase in live weight was 0.40 (±0.05) μm. Secondly, the lower level of nutrition (high stocking rate) increased the medullated fibre content of the fleece from 2.98 to 5.11%.

McGregor (1986) concluded that nutrition and live weight rather than age *per se* are the major determinants of mohair fibre diameter, and that smaller and more poorly fed Angora goats produce finer mohair than larger and better fed Angoras. Although this may apply to adult animals, it should be noted that mean fibre diameter increases markedly as the animal matures, from an average of about 24 μm in kids to around 46 μm in strong adult stock (Westhuysen *et al* 1985).

The pronounced effect that nutrition can have on mohair production is illustrated in the report of Westhuysen *et al* (1985) that supplementary feeding of six-month-old kids during drought conditions more than doubled fibre production over a six-month period.

Mohair production and quality have been shown to respond to both the quantity and degradability of dietary protein. Sahlu *et al* (1988) demonstrated an increase of 23% in clean fleece yield and of 5.25% in mean fibre diameter was associated with an increase in dietary protein from 120 to 180 g/kg. The replacement of solvent-extracted soyabean meal by heat-treated (protected) soyabean meal increased clean fleece yield by 12.6% and mean fibre diameter by 1.8%. Throckmorton *et al* (1982) have also reported increased mohair production following the feeding of formaldehyde-treated casein.

There is little information available on the effect of pre- and post-natal nutrition on skin follicle development, and hence on fibre production, in Angora goats. The secondary follicles are largely initiated by 120 days post-conception and maturation is complete about 4 months after birth (Wentzel and Vosloo 1975, cited by Norton and Ash 1985) and by analogy with work on Merino sheep (Schinckel and Short 1961) nutrition of the dam and the young kid could have important effects on follicle maturation, fibre production and fibre number.

Mohair production is reduced in pregnant and lactating does (Stapleton 1978, cited by Reis 1982) presumably because of competition for essential nutrients between the skin follicles and foetal or mammary tissue. The large fluctuations in mohair price make it difficult for the producer to decide how best to use nutritional effects on fibre quantity and quality to optimise the financial return from mohair production, i.e. whether to feed for the production of an increased weight of coarser fibre or for a lesser quantity of a finer quality mohair.

8.3.2   Cashmere goats

Several workers (e.g. Anon 1983; Johnson and Rowe 1984; Ash and Norton 1984; Russel *pers comm*) have reported that although significant increases in fibre production have been noted in response to increased levels of nutrient input and to the inclusion of higher levels of dietary protein, including proteins of low rumen degradability, these have been wholly attributable to effects on the guard hair. No significant effects of nutrition on the weight of cashmere fibre (secondary follicles) have been reported. Norton and Ash (1985) calculated that less than 0.01 of the total dietary protein intake (CP, g/d) is required to grow a cashmere fleece compared with 0.06 to 0.09 in sheep.

There is some evidence, mostly hearsay, that cashmere quality (i.e. mean fibre diameter) can be influenced by nutrition. Russel (*pers comm*) has shown that undernutrition can significantly reduce the mean fibre diameter of Scottish feral goats from 14.0 to 13.5 µm. Reports that luxury levels of feeding cause coarsening of the fibre have not been substantiated, but may well refer to "cashmere" goats which have some Angora influence in their genetic background. Russel (*pers comm*) found no effect on cashmere weight or mean fibre diameter of the inclusion of 10% fishmeal in a diet fed at 1.67 times maintenance. This accords with the findings of Johnson and Rowe (1984), who concluded that cashmere production does not appear to be dependent on protein supply. When considered in relation to the calculations of Norton and Ash (1985) referred to above, the apparent unresponsiveness of cashmere growth and fibre diameter to nutritional influences may not be unexpected. These workers considered that the primary control of fibre growth in cashmere goats is probably hormonal rather than nutritional.

The work referred to in this section has been conducted largely with feral goats producing relatively small quantities (*circa* 100 g) of cashmere. It remains to be established whether fibre growth might be more responsive to nutrition at higher levels of production (*circa* 400 to 500 g).

Studies on the development of skin follicles in Australian feral goats have shown effects of pre-natal nutrition on the post-natal development of secondary follicles to 4 months of age, but these did not persist beyond that stage (Lambert *et al* 1984). Similarly, early effects of sex and birth type, which are presumed to be mediated through nutritional influences, did not affect the ultimate secondary follicle density. Norton and Ash (1985) concluded that moderate restrictions in either the energy or protein intake of pregnant did do not have any major effect on the pattern or extent of follicle development in their kids. This is supported by the results of McCall and Fitzgerald (1987) which indicate that levels of feeding during late pregnancy and lactation, in most practical situations, are unlikely to influence cashmere production of the progeny.

References

Abrams, E.; Guthrie, P.; Harris, B. (1985) Effect of dry matter intake from whole goat milk and calf milk replacer on performance of Nubian goat kids. *Journal of Dairy Science* **68**, 1748–1751.

Ademosun, A.A.; Munyabantu, C.M. (1982) Copper requirements for the West African dwarf goat. In: *Proceedings of the Third International Conference on Goat Production and Disease,* Scottsdale, Arizona, USA; Dairy Goat Journal Publishing Company, p. 560.

AFRC (1990) Technical Committee on Responses to Nutrients, Report No. 5. Nutritive requirements of ruminant animals: energy. *Nutrition Abstracts & Reviews, Series B* **60**, 729–804.

AFRC (1991) Technical Committee on Responses to Nutrients, Report No. 6. A reappraisal of the calcium and phosphorus requirements of sheep and cattle. *Nutrition Abstracts & Reviews, Series B* **61**, 573–612.

AFRC (1992) Technical Committee on Responses to Nutrients, Report No. 9. Nutritive requirements of ruminant animals: protein. *Nutrition Abstracts & Reviews, Series B* **62**, 787–835.

AFRC (1993) *Energy and protein requirements of ruminants.* Wallingford, UK; CAB International.

Aguilera, J.F.; Prieto, C.; Fonollá, J. (1990) Protein and energy metabolism of lactating Granadina goats. *British Journal of Nutrition* **63**, 165–175.

Akinsoyinu, A.O. (1974) Studies on protein and energy utilization by the West African dwarf goats. *Ph.D. Thesis, University of Ibadan, Nigeria.*

Akinsoyinu, A.O.; Mba, A.U.; Olubajo, F.O. (1975) Studies on energy and protein utilization for pregnancy and lactation by the West African dwarf goats in Nigeria. *East African Agricultural and Forestry Journal* **41**, 167–176.

Akinsoyinu, A.O.; Mba, A.U.; Olubajo, F.O. (1976) Crude protein requirement of West African dwarf goats for maintenance and gain. *Journal of the Association for the Advancement of Agricultural Sciences in Africa* **3**, 75–82.

Alam, M.R.; Poppi, D.P.; Sykes, A.R. (1983) Intake, digestibility and retention time of 2 forages by kids and lambs. *Proceedings of the New Zealand Society of Animal Production* **43**, 119–121.

Alam, M.R.; Poppi, D.P.; Sykes, A.R. (1985) Comparative intake of digestible organic matter and water by sheep and goats. *Proceedings of the New Zealand Society of Animal Production* **45**, 107–111.

Alam, M.R.; Lawson, G.D.; Poppi, D.P.; Sykes, A.R. (1987) Comparison of the site and extent of digestion of nutrients of a forage in kids and lambs. *Journal of Agricultural Science (Cambridge)* **109**, 583–589.

Alam, M.R.; Poppi, D.P.; Sykes, A.R. (1991) Comparative energy and protein utilization in kids and lambs. *Journal of Agricultural Science (Cambridge)* **117**, 121–127.

Alderman, G. (1982) *Provisional nutrient standards for goats.* Nutrition Chemists' Technical Note, Ministry of Agriculture, Fisheries and Food, London, UK; Agricultural Development and Advisory Service, Agricultural Science Service.

Alrahmoun, W.; Bellet, B.; Masson, C.; Tisserand, J.L. (1985) Effets compares du régime alimentaire sur l'activité microbienne dans le rumen des ovins et des caprins. *Reproduction, Nutrition, Developpement* **25**, 757.

Anon (1983) *Avondale Project.* A report to the Kinross Cashmere Company.

Antoniou, T.; Hadjipanayiotou, M. (1985) The digestibility by sheep and goats of five roughages offered alone or with concentrates. *Journal of Agricultural Science (Cambridge)* **105**, 663–671.

ARC (1965) *The nutrient requirements of farm livestock. No.2. Ruminants.* London, UK; Agricultural Research Council.

ARC (1980) *The nutrient requirements of ruminant livestock.* Technical Review by an Agricultural Research Council Working Party, Commonwealth Agriculture Bureau, Farnham Royal, UK.

ARC (1984) *The nutrient requirements of ruminant livestock. Supplement No. 1.* Slough, UK; Commonwealth Agricultural Bureaux.

Argo, C.M.; Smith, J.S. (1983) Relationship of energy requirements and seasonal cycles of food intake in Soay rams. *Journal of Physiology* **343**, 23P–24P.

Armstrong, D.G.; Blaxter, K.L. (1965) Effects of acetic and propionic acids on energy retention and milk secretion in goats. In: *Energy metabolism*, Blaxter, K.L. (Ed.), London, UK; Academic Press, pp. 59–72.

Ash, A.J. (1986) A study of body and cashmere growth in weanling goats. *Ph.D. Thesis, University of Queensland, Australia.*

Ash, A.J.; Norton B.W. (1984) The effect of protein and energy intake on cashmere and body growth of Australian cashmere goats. *Proceedings of the Australian Society of Animal Production* **15**, 247–250.

Ash, A.J.; Norton, B.W. (1987a) Studies with the Australian cashmere goat. I. Growth and digestion in male and female goats given pelleted diets varying in protein content and energy level. *Australian Journal of Agricultural Research* **38**, 957–969.

Ash, A.J.; Norton, B.W. (1987b) Studies with the Australian cashmere goat. II. Effects of dietary protein concentration and feeding level on body composition of male and female goats. *Australian Journal of Agricultural Research* **38**, 971–982.

Badamana, M.S. (1987) Forage utilization by dairy goats. *Ph.D. Thesis, University of Reading, UK.*

Badamana, M.S.; Sutton, J.D. (1987) The effect of level of protein in the concentrates on hay intake, milk production and digestive processes by Saanen goats. *Animal Production* **44**, 496.

Badamana, M.S.; Sutton, J.D.; Oldham, J.D.; Mowlem, A. (1990) The effect of amount of protein in the concentrates on hay intake and rate of passage, diet digestibility and milk production in British Saanen goats. *Animal Production* **51**, 333–342.

Bell, H.M. (1973) *Rangeland management for livestock production.* Norman, Oklahoma, USA: University of Oklahoma Press.

Bines, J.A.; Suzuki, S.; Balch, C.C. (1969) The quantitative significance of long-term regulation of food intake in the cow. *British Journal of Nutrition* **23**, 695–704.

Blanchart, G.; Brun-Bellut, J.; Vignon, B. (1980) Comparaison des caprins aux ovins quant a l'ingestion, la digestibilité et la valeur alimentaire de diverses rations. *Reproduction, Nutrition, Developpement* **20**, 1731–1737.

Blaxter, K.L. (1962) *The energy metabolism of ruminants.* London, UK; Hutchinson.

Blaxter, K.L.; Boyne, A.W. (1970) A new method of expressing the nutritive value of feeds as sources of energy. In: *Energy metabolism of farm animals*, Schurch, A.; Wenk, C. (Eds). Juris Druck, Zurich, pp. 9–13.

Blaxter, K.L.; Boyne, A.W. (1982) Fasting and maintenance metabolism of sheep. *Journal of Agricultural Science (Cambridge)* **99**, 611–620.

Bosworth, A.W.; Van Slyke, L.L. (1916) The soluble and insoluble compounds of goat's milk. *Journal of Biological Chemistry* **24**, 177.

Brett, D.J.; Corbett, J.L.; Inskip, M.W. (1972) Estimation of the energy value of ewe milk. *Proceedings of the Australian Society of Animal Production* **9**, 286–291.

Brody, S. (1945) *Bioenergetics and growth.* 1974 reprint, New York, USA; Hafner Press.

Brown, D.L.; Taylor, S.J. (1986) Deuterium oxide dilution kinetics to predict body composition in dairy goats. *Journal of Dairy Science* **69**, 1151–1155.

Brun-Bellut, J. (1986) Détermination des besoins azotés de la chèvre en lactation. *Thesis, Institut National Polytechnique de Lorraine, France* (Cited by Brun-Bellut *et al* 1987).

Brun-Bellut, J.; Blanchart, G.; Vignon, B. (1984) Détermination des besoins azotés de la chèvre en lactation. *Annales de Zootechnie* **33**, 171–185.

Brun-Bellut, J.; Blanchart, G.; Laurent, F.; Vignon, B. (1987) Nitrogen requirement for goats. In: *Proceedings of the IV International Conference on Goats, Vol. 2*, Santana, O.P.; Silva, A.G. da; Foote, W.C. (Eds), Brasilia, Brazil; EMBRAPA-DDT, pp. 1205–1223.

Cabrera, R.; Villarroel, P.; Vial, E.; Castillo, A. (1983) Rumen fermentative activity in the goat and sheep. *South African Journal of Animal Science* **13**, 213–215.

Castle, E.J. (1956) The rate of passage of foodstuffs through the alimentary tract of the goat. 1. Studies on adult animals fed on hay and concentrates. *British Journal of Nutrition* **10**, 15–23.

Chhabra, A.; Arora, S.P. (1985) Effect of zinc deficiency on serum vitamin A level, tissue enzymes and histological alterations in goats. *Livestock Production Science* **12**, 69–77.

Chilliard, Y. (1985) Métabolisme de tissus adipeux, lipogénèse mammaire et activités lipoprotéine-lipasiques chez la chèvre au cours du cycle gestation-lactation. *Ph.D. Thesis, Université Pierre et Marie Curie, Paris, France* (Cited by Morand-Fehr *et al* 1987).

Ciszuk, P. (1980) Nitrogen balance and digestibility in lactating goats on rations with varied nitrogen and energy sources. *Report 53, Swedish University of Agricultural Sciences, Uppsala, Sweden.*

Ciszuk, P.; Lindberg, J.E. (1985) Total nitrogen retention in lactating goats in relation to digested nitrogen and estimated absorption of amino acids. *Acta Agriculturæ Scandinavica* Supplement 25, pp. 163–176.

Ciszuk, P.; Lindberg, J.E. (1988) Responses in feed intake, digestibility and nitrogen retention in lactating dairy goats fed increasing amounts of urea and fish meal. *Acta Agriculturæ Scandinavica* **38**, 381–395.

Clark, D.A.; Lambert, M.G.; Rolston, M.P.; Dymock, N. (1982) Diet selection by goats and sheep on hill country. *Proceedings of the New Zealand Society of Animal Production* **42**, 155–157.

Collins, H.A.; Nicol, A.M. (1986) The consequences for feed dry matter intake of grazing sheep, cattle and goats to the same residual herbage mass. *Proceedings of the New Zealand Society of Animal Production* **46**, 125–128.

Cowan, R.T.; Robinson, J.J.; Greenhalgh, J.F.D.; McHattie, I. (1979) Body composition changes in lactating ewes estimated by serial slaughter and deuterium dilution. *Animal Production* **29**, 81–90.

Cowan, R.T.; Robinson, J.J.; McDonald, I.; Smart, R. (1980) Effects of body fatness at lambing and diet in lactation on body tissue loss, feed intake and milk yield of ewes in early lactation. *Journal of Agricultural Science (Cambridge)* **95**, 497–514.

Cowan, R.T.; Robinson, J.J.; McHattie, I.; Pennie, K. (1981) Effects of protein concentration in the diet on milk yield, change in body composition and the efficiency of utilization of body tissue for milk production in ewes. *Animal Production* **33**, 111–120.

CVB (1991) *Veevoedertabel.* Lelystad, Netherlands; Centraal Veevoederbureau in Nederlands.

De Jong, A. (1981) A short and long term effect of eating on blood composition in free-feeding goats. *Journal of Agricultural Science (Cambridge)* **96**, 659–668.

Devendra, C. (1967) Studies in the nutrition of the indigenous goat of Malaya. II. The maintenance requirement of pen-fed goat. *Malaysian Agricultural Journal* **46**, 80–97.

Devendra, C. (1978) The digestive efficiency of goats. *World Review of Animal Production* **14**, 9–22.

Devendra, C. (1980) The protein requirements for maintenance of indigenous Kambing Katjang goats in Malaysia. *Malaysian Agricultural Research and Development Institute Research Bulletin* 8, 111–126.

Devendra, C.; Burns, M. (1983) *Goat production in the tropics.* 2nd Edition. Slough, UK; Commonwealth Agricultural Bureaux.

Domingue, B.M.F.; Dellow, D.W.; Barry, T.N. (1991) Voluntary intake and rumen digestion of low-quality roughage by goats and sheep. *Journal of Agricultural Science* **117**, 111–120.

Doyle, P.T.; Egan, J.K. (1980) Intake and digestion of herbage diets by Angora goats and Merino sheep. *Proceedings of the Australian Society of Animal Production* **13**, 521.

Dunshea, F.R.; Bell, A.W.; Trigg, T.E. (1990) Body composition changes in goats during early lactation estimated using a two-pool model of tritiated water kinetics. *British Journal of Nutrition* **64**, 121–131.

Economides, S. (1986) Comparative studies of sheep and goats: milk yield and composition and growth rate of lambs and kids. *Journal of Agricultural Science (Cambridge)* **106**, 477–484.

Eriksson, S.; Sanne, S.; Thomke S. (1976) *Fodermedelstabeller och Utfodringsrekommendationer,* 2nd Edition. LTS Förlag, Stockholm.

Flatt, W.P.; Moe, P.W.; Moore, L.A.; Breirem, K.; Ekern, A. (1972) Energy requirements in lactation. In: *Handbuch der Tierernährung, Vol. 2,* Lenkeit, W.; Breirem, K.; Crasemann, E. (Eds), Hamburg, Germany; Verlag Paul Parey, pp. 341–392.

Forbes, J.M. (1986) *The voluntary food intake of farm animals.* London, UK; Butterworths.

French, M.H. (1970) Observations on the goat. *FAO Agricultural Studies No. 80. FAO Animal Production and Health Series No. 14.* Rome, Italy; Food and Agriculture Organisation of the United Nations.

Fujihara, T.; Tasaki, I.; Furuhasi, T. (1973) Energetic utilization of starch introduced into abomasum of goats. In: *Energy metabolism of farm animals, Proceedings of 6th Symposium on Energy Metabolism,* Menke, K.H.; Lantsch, H.-J.; Reichl, J.R. (Eds), Stuttgart, Germany; University of Hohenheim, pp. 67–70.

Gamble, A.W.; Mackintosh, J.B. (1982) A comparison of digestion in goats and sheep of similar live weights. *Proceedings of the Australian Society of Animal Production* **14**, 652.

Gentry, A.W. (1978) In: *Evolution of African mammals,* Maglio, V.J.; Cooke, H.B.S. (Eds), London, UK; Harvard University Press, p. 536.

Gibb, M.J.; Ivings, W.E.; Dhanoa, M.S.; Sutton, J.D. (1992) Changes in body components of autumn-calving Holstein-Friesian cows over the first 29 weeks of lactation. *Animal Production* **55**, 339–360.

Gibb, M.J.; Cook, J.E.; Treacher, T.T. (1993) Performance of British Saanen, Boer x British Saanen and Anglo-Nubian castrated male kids from 8 weeks to slaughter at 28, 33 or 38 kg liveweight. *Animal Production* **57**, 263–271.

Giger, S. (1987) Influence de la composition de l'aliment concentré sur la valeur alimentaire des rations destinées au ruminant laitier. *Ph.D. Thesis, INA-PG, France* (Cited by Morand-Fehr *et al* 1987).

Gihad, E.A. (1979) Intake, digestibility and nutrient utilization by sheep of sodium hydroxide-treated tropical grass supplemented with soyabean or urea. *Journal of Animal Science* **48**, 1172–1176.

Goatcher, W.D.; Church, D.C. (1970) Taste responses in ruminants. IV. Reactions of pygmy goats, normal goats, sheep and cattle to acetic acid and quinine hydrochloride. *Journal of Animal Science* **31**, 373–382.

Grant, S.A.; Bolton, G.R.; Russel, A.J.F. (1984) The utilization of sown and indigenous plant species by sheep and goats grazing hill pastures. *Grass and Forage Science* **39**, 361–370.

Gueguen, L.; Lamand, M.; Meschy, F. (1988) Nutrition minerale. In: *Alimentation des bovins, ovins and caprins,* Jarrige, R. (Ed.), Paris, France; Institut National de la Recherche Agronomique, pp. 95–111.

Guerrero, J.E. (1982) Estudio de la alimentación del ganado caprino. Utilización de subproductos y ensayos de lactación en cabras de raza Granadina. *Ph.D. Thesis, University of Cordoba, Spain* (Cited by Aguilera *et al* 1990).

Guss, S.B. (1977) *Management and diseases of dairy goats.* Scottsdale, Arizona, USA; Dairy Goat Journal Publishing Company.

Hadjipanayiotou, M.; Antoniou, T. (1983) A comparison of rumen fermentation patterns in sheep and goats given a variety of diets. *Journal of the Science of Food and Agriculture* **34**, 1319–1322.

Hadjipanayiotou, M.; Georghiades, E.; Koumas, A. (1988a) The effect of protein source on the performance of suckling Chios ewes and Damascus goats. *Animal Production* **46**, 249–255.

Hadjipanayiotou, M.; Koumas, A.; Georghiades, E.; Hadjidemetriou, D. (1988b) Studies on degradation and outflow rate of protein supplements in the rumen of dry and lactating Chios ewes and Damascus goats. *Animal Production* **46**, 243–248.

Haenlein, G.F.W. (1980a) Nutrient requirements of dairy goats – past and present. *International Goat and Sheep Research* **1**, 79–95.

Haenlein, G.F.W. (1980b) Mineral nutrition of goats. *Journal of Dairy Science* **63**, 1729–1748.

Haenlein, G.F.W. (1984) Dietary nutrient allowances for goats and sheep. *Feedstuffs* **56**, 68–71.

Haenlein, G.F.W. (1987) Mineral and vitamin requirements and deficiencies. In: *Proceedings of the IV International Conference on Goats, Vol. 2,* Santana, O.P.; Silva, A.G. da; Foote, W.C. (Eds), Brasilia, Brazil; EMBRAPA-DDT, pp. 1249–1266.

Hafez, E.S.E. (1975) *The behaviour of domestic animals.* 3rd Edition. London, UK; Bailliere Tindall.

Havrevoll, Ø. (1985) Bucket feeding and teat feeding of acidified or non-acidified milk feed for rearing dairy goats. *Annales de Zootechnie* **34**, 486–487.

Havrevoll, Ø.; Garmo, G.; Hellberghausen, O.; Solheim, J. (1985) *Forsok med botteforing og Smokkforing av sott og surna mjolkefor til geitkje. Meldinger fra Norges Lanbrukshogskole* **64**, 15.

Hines, T.G.; Horst, R.L.; Littledike, E.T.; Beitz, D.C.; Jacobson, N.L. (1986a) Vitamin D3 and D3 metabolites in young goats fed varying amounts of calcium and vitamin D3. *Journal of Dairy Science* **69**, 385–391.

Hines, T.G.; Jacobson, N.L.; Beitz, D.C.; Littledike, E.T. (1986b) Effects of dietary calcium, vitamin D3 and corn supplementation on growth performance and mineral metabolism in young goats fed whole milk diets. *Journal of Dairy Science* **69**, 2868–2876.

Holmes, A.D.; Kuzmeski, J.W.; Lindquist, H.G.; Rodman, H.B. (1946) Goat's milk as a source of bone building minerals for infant feeding. *American Journal of Diseases of Children* **71**, 647.

Howe, J.C.; Barry, T.N.; Popay, A.I. (1988) Voluntary intake and digestion of gorse (*Ulex europaeus*) by goats and sheep. *Journal of Agricultural Science (Cambridge)* **111,** 107–114.

Humphries, W.R.; Morrice, P.C.; Mitchell, A.N. (1987) Copper poisoning in Angora goats. *Veterinary Record* **121**, 231.

Huston, J.E. (1978) Forage utilization and nutrient requirements of the goat. *Journal of Dairy Science* **61**, 988–993.

IDWP (1984) Mineral, trace element and vitamin allowances for ruminant livestock. MAFF, DAFS, DANI, UKASTA and BVA, Report of an Interdepartmental Working Party. In: *Recent advances in animal nutrition – 1984,* Haresign, W.; Cole, D.J.A (Eds), London, UK; Butterworths, pp. 113–142.

INRA (1978) *Alimentation des ruminants.* Versailles, France; Institut National de la Recherche Agronomique.

INRA (1988) *Alimentation des bovins, ovins et caprins.* Paris, France; Institut National de la Recherche Agronomique.

Islay and Jura Goat Society (1985) *Goat Husbandry Survey Report.* Argyll, Isle of Islay, UK; Islay and Jura Goat Society.

Itoh, M.; Haryu, T.; Tano, R.; Iwasaki, K. (1977) Maintenance requirements of energy and protein for castrated Japanese native goats. *Bulletin of National Institute of Animal Industry (Japan), No. 33,* 41–50.

Jagusch, K.T.; Kidd, G.T. (1982) In: *Seminar on Dairy Goat Husbandry and Medicine,* Northland Branch NZVA, Whangare, New Zealand.

Jagusch, K.T.; Duganzich, D.M.; Kidd, G.T.; Church, S.M. (1983) Efficiency of goat milk utilization by milk-fed kids. *New Zealand Journal of Agricultural Research* **26,** 443–445.

Jarrige, R.; Demarquilly, C.; Dulphy, J.P.; Hoden, A.; Robelin, J.; Beranger, C.; Geay, Y.; Journet, M.; Malterre, C.; Micol, D.; Petit, M. (1986) The INRA "fill unit" system for predicting the voluntary intake of forage-based diets in ruminants: a review. *Journal of Animal Science* **63,** 1737–1758.

Jenness, R. (1980) Composition and characteristics of goat milk: review 1968–1979. *Journal of Dairy Science* **63,** 1605–1630.

Johnson, T.J.; Rowe, J.B. (1984) Growth and cashmere production by goats in relation to dietary protein supply. *Proceedings of the Australian Society of Animal Production* **15,** 400–403.

Kameoka, K.; Morimoto, H. (1959) Extent of digestion in the rumen-reticulum-omasum of goats. *Journal of Dairy Science* **42,** 1187–1197.

Kearl, L.C. (1982) *Nutrient requirements of ruminants in developing countries.* Utah State University, Logan, USA; International Feedstuffs Institute.

Kessler, J. (1981) Éléments minéraux majeurs chez la chèvre données de base et apports recommandés. In: *Nutrition and systems of goat feeding, Vol. I,* Morand-Fehr, P.; Bourbouze, A.; Simiane, M. de (Eds), Paris, France; ITOVIC-INRA, pp. 196–209.

Kessler, J. (1984) Apports recommandés pour les caprins. In: *Apports alimentaires recommandés et tables de la valeur nutritive des aliments pour les ruminants,* 2nd Edition, Schneeberger, H.; Landis, J. (Eds), Zollikofen, Switzerland; Centrale des moyens d'enseignement agricole, pp. 89–105.

Kessler, J. (1987) Effect of a high dietary potassium content on Mg-, K-, and Na-metabolism in the lactating goat. *Annales de Zootechnie* **36,** 319–344.

Kessler, J.; Wanner, M.; Gubler, D.; Schneeberger, H. (1986) Effect of a parenteral dose of vitamin E and selenium on vitamin E/selenium status of goats and kids. *Journal of Animal Physiology and Animal Nutrition* **56,** 41–51.

Knowles, F.; Watkin, J.E. (1938) The milk of the goat under English conditions. *Journal of Dairy Research* **9,** 153–165.

Konar, A.; Thomas, P.C.; Rook, J.A.F. (1971) The concentrations of some water-soluble constituents in the milk of cows, sows, ewes and goats. *Journal of Dairy Research* **38,** 333–341.

Lachica, M.; Prieto, C.; Aguilera, J.F. (1997) The energy cost of walking on the level and on negative and postive slopes in the Granadina goat (*Capra hircus*). *British Journal of Nutrition* **77,** 73–81.

Lamand, M. (1981) Métabolisme et besoins en oligo-éléments des chèvres. In: *Nutrition and systems of goat feeding, Vol. 1,* Morand-Fehr, P.; Bourbouze, A.; Simiane, M. de (Eds), Paris, France; ITOVIC-INRA, pp. 210–217.

Lambert, A.; Restall, B.J.; Norton, B.W.; Winter, J.D. (1984) The post natal development of hair follicle groups in the skin of the Australian feral goat. *Proceedings of the Australian Society of Animal Production* **15,** 420–423.

Laurent, F.; Blanchart, J.; Brun-Bellut, J. (1987) Nitrogen flows in the gut of dairy goats: quantitative and qualitative aspects. *Annales de Zootechnie* **36**, 327–328.

Lindahl, I.L. (1955) Goat feeding investigations. *Annual Report, Animal and poultry husbandry research branch, Agricultural Research Service, US Department of Agriculture* (Cited by Morand-Fehr and Sauvant 1978).

Lindahl, I.L. (1956) Goat feeding investigations. *Annual Report, Animal and poultry husbandry research branch, Agricultural Research Service, US Department of Agriculture* (Cited by Morand-Fehr and Sauvant 1978).

Linzell, J.L. (1967) The effect of very frequent milking and of oxytocin on the yield and composition of milk in fed and fasted goats. *Journal of Physiology* **190**, 333.

Lu, C.D. (1988) Grazing behaviour and diet selection of goats. *Small Ruminant Research* **1**, 205–216.

Lu, C.D.; Coleman, L.J. (1986) Grazing behaviour and diet selection of goats. In: *Proceedings of the 1st Regional Goat Conference*. Tallahassee, Florida, USA; Florida A and M University, p. 56.

Lu, C.D.; Iglesias, T.I.; Nelson, R.R.; Rubin, J.L.; Teh, T.H. (1984) Response of lactating dairy goats to dietary protein and energy levels. *Journal of Dairy Science* **67**, Supplement No. 1, 132–133.

Madsen, J. (1985) The basis for the Nordic protein evaluation system for ruminants. The AAT/PBV system. *Acta Agriculturæ Scandinavica* Supplement 25, 9–20.

Majumdar, B.N. (1960a) Studies on goat nutrition. I. Minimum protein requirement of goats for maintenance. Endogenous urinary nitrogen and metabolic faecal nitrogen excretion studies. *Journal of Agricultural Science (Cambridge)* **54**, 329–334.

Majumdar, B.N. (1960b) Studies on goat nutrition. II. Digestible protein requirements for maintenance from balance studies. *Journal of Agricultural Science (Cambridge)* **54**, 335–340.

Maraval, B.; Vignon, B. (1982) Entwicklung der Mineralzusammensetzung von Ziegenmilch zu Beginn der Laktation. *Milchwissenschaft* **37**, 464–466.

Mason, V.C. (1969) Some observations on the distribution and origin of nitrogen in sheep faeces. *Journal of Agricultural Science (Cambridge)* **73**, 99–111.

Masson, C.; Alrahmoun, W.; Tisserand, J.L. (1986) A comparative study of feed intake, digestibility, nitrogen utilization, mean retention time and feeding behaviour of young goats and sheep fed on different diets. *Annales de Zootechnie* **35**, 49–59.

Mavrogenis, A.P.; Papachristoforou, C. (1988) Estimation of the energy value of milk and prediction of fat-corrected milk yield in sheep and goats. *Small Ruminant Research* **1**, 229–236.

Mba, A.U. (1982) Mineral nutrition of goats in Nigeria. In: *Proceedings of the Third International Conference on Goat Production and Disease*, Scottsdale, Arizona, USA; Dairy Goat Journal Publishing Company, pp. 109–112.

McCall, D.G.; Fitzgerald, J.M. (1987) Growth and fleece responses of cashmere goats to late pregnancy and lactation feeding at pasture. *Proceedings of the Second International Cashmere Conference*, p. 125.

McCall, D.G.; Lambert, M.G. (1987) Pasture feeding of goats. In: *Livestock feeding on pasture*, Occasional Publication No. 10, New Zealand Society of Animal Production, p. 105.

McCammon-Feldman, B.; Van Soest, P.J.; Horvath, P.; McDowell, R.E. (1981) Feeding strategy of the goat. *Cornell International Agriculture Mimeograph No 88*, Ithaca, New York, USA; Cornell University.

McDonald, I.; Robinson, J.J.; Fraser, C.; Smart, R.I. (1979) Studies on reproduction in prolific ewes. 5. The accretion of nutrients in the foetuses and adnexas. *Journal of Agricultural Science (Cambridge)* **92**, 591–603.

McGregor, B.A. (1984) Growth and fleece production of Angora wethers grazing annual pastures. *Proceedings of the Australian Society of Animal Production* **15**, 715.

McGregor, B.A. (1986) Liveweight and nutritional influences on fibre diameter of mohair. *Proceedings of the Australian Society of Animal Production* **16**, 420.

McMahon, C.A. (1964) Comparative food habits of deer and three classes of livestock. *Journal of Wildlife Management* **28**, 798–808.

Merrill, L.B.; Taylor, C.A. (1981) Diet selection, grazing habits, and the place of goats in range management. In: *Goat production,* Gall, C. (Ed.), London, UK; Academic Press, pp. 233–252.

Mohammed, H.H. (1982) Energy requirements for maintenance and growth: comparison of goats and sheep. *Ph.D. Thesis, University of Reading, UK.*

Mohammed, H.H.; Owen, E. (1981) Comparison of the maintenance energy requirement of sheep and goats fed dried lucerne and dried grass. In: *Nutrition and systems of goat feeding, Vol. 2,* Morand-Fehr, P.; Bourbouze, A.; Simiane, M. de (Eds), Paris, France; ITOVIC-INRA, pp. 18–22.

Mohammed, H.H.; Owen, E. (1982) Goats versus sheep: effect of coat thickness and body composition on maintenance energy requirement. *Animal Production* **43**, 391.

Morand-Fehr, P. (1981) Nutrition and feeding of goats: application to temperate climatic conditions. In: *Goat production,* Gall, C. (Ed.), London, UK; Academic Press, pp. 193–232.

Morand-Fehr, P.; Sauvant, D. (1978a) Caprins. In: *Alimentation des ruminants,* Jarrige, R. (Ed.), Versailles, France; Institut National de la Recherche Agronomique, pp. 449–467.

Morand-Fehr, P.; Sauvant, D. (1978b) Nutrition and optimum performance of dairy goats. *Livestock Production Science* **5**, 203–213.

Morand-Fehr, P.; Sauvant, D. (1980) Composition and yield of goat milk as affected by nutritional manipulation. *Journal of Dairy Science* **63**, 1671–1680.

Morand-Fehr, P.; Sauvant, D. (1988) Alimentation des caprins. In: *Alimentation des bovins, ovins et caprins,* Jarrige, R. (Ed.), Paris, France; Institut National de la Recherche Agronomique, pp. 282–304.

Morand-Fehr, P.; Hervieu, J.; Bas, P.; Sauvant D. (1982) *Proceedings of the Third International Conference on Goat Production and Disease,* Scottsdale, Arizona, USA; Dairy Goat Journal Publishing Company, pp. 90–104.

Morand-Fehr, P.; Blanchart, G.; Le Mens, P.; Remeuf, F.; Sauvant, D.; Lenoir, J.; Lamberet, G.; Le Jaouen, J.C.; Bas, P. (1986) Données recentes sur la composition du lait de chèvre. *Journées de la Recherche Ovine et Caprine* **11**, 253–298.

Morand-Fehr, P.; Sauvant, D.; Brun-Bellut, J. (1987) Recommandations alimentaires pour les caprins. *Bulletin Technique, C.R.Z.V. Theix* **70**, 213–222.

Morgen, A.; Beger, C.; Fingerling, G. (1906) Weitere Untersuchungen über die Wirkung einzelnen Nährstoffe und die Milchproduktion. *Landwirtschaftliche Versuchsstationen* **64**, 93–242 (Cited by Haenlein 1980).

Mowlem, A. (1972) Breeding goats for research. *Journal of the Institute of Animal Technicians* **23**, 125–135.

Mowlem, A. (1979) Milk replacers for kid rearing. *British Goat Society Yearbook*, pp. 54–57.

Mowlem, A. (1984) Artificial rearing of kids. *Goat Veterinary Society Journal* 5, 25–30.

Mowlem, A. (1985) The use of milk replacers based on soya protein and whey for kid rearing. *Annales de Zootechnie* 34, 485.

Mowlem, A. (1988) *Goat farming*. Ipswich, UK; Farming Press Books.

Naate, N.M. (1986) Effect of the level of offer on selection and intake of barley straw by sheep. *M.Phil. Thesis, University of Reading, UK*.

Naga, M.A.; Nour, A.M.; Borhami, B.E.; El-din, M.Z.; Abaza, M.A.; El-Shazley, K.; Abou Akkada, A.R.; Oltjen, R.R. (1978) Effect of potassium on the rumen microorganisms of animals fed on diets containing urea. *Tropical Animal Production* 3, 62–68.

Ndosa, J.E.M. (1980) A comparative study of roughage utilisation by sheep and goats. *M.Phil. Thesis, University of Reading, UK*.

Nitzan, Z.; Carasso, Y.; Nir, I. (1985) The use of starch and soybean protein in intensive rearing of veal-type kids. *Annales de Zootechnie* 34, 487–488.

Norton, B.W.; Ash, A.J. (1985) Recent advances in goat nutrition in Australia. In: *Recent advances in animal nutrition in Australia,* Cumming, R.B. (Ed.), Armidale, Australia; University of New England, Paper No. 37.

NRC (1981) Nutrient requirements of goats. Angora, dairy and meat goat in temperate and tropical countries. In: *Nutrient requirements of domestic animals, Number 15.* Washington DC, USA; National Academy Press.

NRC (1985a) *Ruminant nitrogen usage.* Washington DC, USA; US National Academy of Science.

NRC (1985b) *Nutrient requirements for sheep.* 6th Revised Edition. Washington DC, USA; National Academy Press.

Oldham, J.D.; Mowlem, A.; Nash, S.J. (1983) Barley straw v. hay for British Saanen goats in late pregnancy and in lactation. In: *Report, 1982, National Institute for Research in Dairying, Shinfield, Reading,* UK, p. 130.

Oldham, J.D.; Mowlem, A.; Nash, S.J. (1984) Effect of concentrate allowance on performance of lactating Saanen goats. In: *Report, 1983, National Institute for Research in Dairying, Shinfield, Reading,* UK, pp. 102–103.

Oldham, J.D.; Mowlem, A.; Nash, S.J. (1985) Effect of concentrate allowance on performance of lactating Saanen goats. In: *Report, 1984–5, National Institute for Research in Dairying, Shinfield, Reading,* UK, pp. 169–170.

Opstvedt, J. (1967) Feeding experiments with goats. I. Studies on the effect of energy level and feed combination on feed intake and milk yield, composition and organoleptic properties. *Bull. Techn. No. 134, Agricultural College of Norway.*

Orr, J.B.; Magee, H.E. (1923) The use of indirect calorimetry in ruminants. *Journal of Agricultural Science (Cambridge)* 13, 447–461.

Ørskov, E.R.; McDonald, I. (1979) The estimation of protein degradability in the rumen from incubation measurements weighted according to rate of passage. *Journal of Agricultural Science* 92, 499–503.

Ørskov, E.R.; Mehrez, A.Z. (1977) Estimation of extent of protein degradation from basal feeds in the rumen of sheep. *Proceedings of the Nutrition Society* 36, 78A.

Ørskov, E.R.; Grubb, D.A.; Wenham, G.; Corrigall, W. (1979) The sustenance of growing and fattening ruminants by intragastric infusion of volatile fatty acid and protein. *British Journal of Nutrition* **41**, 553–558.

Owen, E.; de Paiva, P. (1980) Artificial rearing of goat kids: effect of age at weaning and milk substitute restriction on performance to slaughter weight. *Animal Production* **30**, 480.

Panaretto, B.A. (1963) Body composition *in vivo*. III. The composition of living ruminants and its relation to the tritiated water spaces. *Australian Journal of Agricultural Research* **14**, 944–952.

Panaretto, B.A.; Till, A.R. (1963) Body composition *in vivo*. II. The composition of mature goats and its relationship to the antipyrine, tritiated water, and N-acetyl-4-aminoantipyrine spaces. *Australian Journal of Agricultural Research* **14**, 926–943.

Pant, H.C.; Rawat, J.S.; Roy, A. (1962) Studies on rumen physiology, 1. Growth of fistulated animals and standardisation of methods. *Indian Journal of Dairy Science* **15**, 167–185.

Parkash, S.; Jenness, R. (1968) The composition and characteristics of goats' milk: a review. *Dairy Science Abstracts* **30**, 67–87.

Prieto, C.; Aguilera, J.F.; Lara, L.; Fonollá, J. (1990) Protein and energy requirements for maintenance of indigenous Granadina goats. *British Journal of Nutrition* **63**, 155–163.

Prieto, C.; Lachica, M.; Garcia-Barroso, F.; Aguilera, J.F.; Boza, J. (1991) The effect of seasonal variation in the grazing activities on the energy requirements of goats. *FAO Network of Cooperative Research on Sheep and Goats. Proceedings of the Subnetwork Nutrition*, Lindberg, J.E. (Ed.), Östersund, Sweden; Sverige Lantbruksuniversitet, pp. 20–21.

Prieto,C.; Sanz Sampelayo, M.R.; Gil Extremera, F.; Boza, J. (1993) Feed intake and performance in pre-ruminant kid goats and lambs at different environmental temperatures. In: *FAO-CIHEAM-EC Meeting on Sheep and Goat Nutrition*, Thessaloniki, Greece; Aristotle University of Thessaloniki, p. 21.

Radcliffe, J.E. (1982) Gorse control with sheep and goats. In: *Proceedings of the 35th New Zealand Weed and Pest Control Conference*, Hartley, M.J. (Ed.), Palmerston North, New Zealand; New Zealand Weed and Pest Control Society Inc., pp. 130–134.

Rajpoot, R.L. (1978) Energy and protein in goat nutrition. *Ph.D. Thesis, Department of Animal Husbandry, Dairy R.B.S. College Bichpuri, India.*

Rajpoot, R.L.; Sengar, O.P.S.; Singh, S.N. (1980) Goats: protein requirement for maintenance. *International Goat and Sheep Research* **1**, 182–189 (Cited by Brun-Bellut *et al* 1984).

Randy, H.A.; Sniffen, C.J.; Heintz, J.F. (1988) Effect of age and stage of lactation on dry matter intake and milk production in Alpine does. *Small Ruminant Research* **1**, 145–149.

Reis, P.J. (1982) Growth and characteristics of wool and hair. In: *Sheep and goat production,* Coop, I.E. (Ed.), Amsterdam, Netherlands; Elsevier.

Reynolds, L. (1981) Nitrogen metabolism in indigenous Malawi goats. *Journal of Agricultural Science (Cambridge)* **96**, 347–351.

Ritzman, E.G.; Washburn, L.E.; Benedict, F.G. (1936) The basal metabolism of the goat. *New Hampshire Agricultural Experiment Station Technical Bulletin 66.*

Robinson, J.J.; McDonald, I.; Fraser, C.; Crofts, R.M.J. (1977) Studies on reproduction in prolific ewes. I. Growth of the products of conception. *Journal of*

Agricultural Science (Cambridge) **88**, 539–552.

Rolston, M.P.; Lambert, M.G.; Clark, D.A.; Devantier, B.P. (1981) Control of rushes and thistles in pastures by goat and sheep grazing. In: *Proceedings of the 34th New Zealand Weed and Pest Control Conference*, pp. 117–121.

Roy-Smith, F. (1980) The fasting metabolism and relative energy intake of goats compared with sheep. *Animal Production* **30**, 491.

Russel, A.J.F.; Adkins, J.E. (1990) Production and composition of milk from suckled feral, dairy and crossbred goats. *Animal Production*, **50**, 565.

Russel, A.J.F.; Maxwell, T.J.; Bolton, G.R.; Currie, D.C.; White, I.R. (1983) A note on the possible use of goats in hill sheep grazing systems. *Animal Production* **36**, 313–316.

Sahlu, T.; Fernandez, J.H.; Manning, R. (1988) Dietary protein degradability and mohair production. In: *Proceedings of the Third Annual Field Day of the American Institute for Goat Research*. Oklahoma, USA; Langston University, pp. 81–84.

Sanz Sampelayo, M.R.; Munoz, F.J.; Guerrero, J.E.; Gil Extremera, F.; Boza, J. (1988) Energy metabolism of the Granadina breed goat kid. Use of goat milk and a milk replacer. *Journal of Animal Physiology and Animal Nutrition* **59**, 1–9.

Sanz Sampelayo, M.R.; Ruiz, I.; Gil, F.; Boza, J. ((1990) Body composition of goat kids during sucking. Voluntary feed intake. *British Journal of Nutrition* **64**, 611–617.

Sauvant, D. (1981) Alimentation energetique des caprins. In: *Nutrition and systems of goat feeding*. Morand-Fehr, P.; Bourbouze, A.; Simiane, M. de (Eds), Paris, France; ITOVIC-INRA, pp. 55–79.

Sauvant, D.; Morand-Fehr, P. (1991) Energy requirements and allowances of adult goats. In: *Goat nutrition*, Morand-Fehr, P. (Ed.), Pudoc, Wageningen, pp. 61–72.

Sauvant, D.; Chilliard, Y.; Morand-Fehr, P. (1991) Etiological aspects of nutritional and metabolic disorders of goats. In: *Goat nutrition*, Morand-Fehr, P. (Ed.), Wageningen, Netherlands; Pudoc, pp. 124–142.

SCA (1990) *Feeding standards for Australian livestock*. Standing Committee of Agriculture, Ruminants Sub-Committee. CSIRO Publications, Melbourne, Australia.

Schinckel, P.G.; Short, B.F. (1961) The influence of nutritional level during pre-natal and early post-natal life on adult fleece and body characters. *Australian Journal of Agricultural Research* **12**, 176.

Sengar, O.P.S. (1980) Indian research on protein and energy requirements of goats. *Journal of Dairy Science* **63**, 1655–1670.

Sibanda, L.M.; Mkumbo, G.; Sutton, J.D.; Owen, E. (1989) Intake of straw, alkali-treated straw and hay by Saanen goats in mid lactation. *Animal Production* **48**, 653.

Simiane, M. de; Giger, S.; Blanchart, G.; Huguet, L. (1981) Valeur nutritionnelle et utilisation des fourrages cultivés intensivement. In: *Nutrition and systems of goat feeding, Vol. 1*, Morand-Fehr, P.; Bourbouze, A.; Simiane, M. de (Eds), Paris, France; ITOVIC-INRA, pp. 274–299.

Simpson, G.G. (1945) *The principles of classification and a classification of mammals*. Bulletin of the American Museum of Natural History, New York, **85**, 1.

Singh, S.N.; Sengar, O.P.S. (1978) Investigation on milk and meat potentialities of Indian goats. *Final Technical Report P.L. 480, Research Project No. A7 – AH – 18, R.B.S. College Bichpuri, India*.

Skjevdal, T. (1974) Potatoes and swedes in the diet of ruminants. III. Studies in lactating dairy goats. *Agricultural University of Norway, Department of Animal Production Report No. 169*, 42 pp.

Skjevdal, T. (1981) Effect on goat performances of given quantities of feedstuffs, and their planned distribution during the cycle of reproduction. In: *Nutrition and systems of goat feeding, Vol. 1*, Morand-Fehr, P.; Bourbouze, A.; Simiane, M. de (Eds) Paris, France; ITOVIC-INRA, pp. 300–318.

Skjevdal, T. (1982) Nutrient requirements of dairy goats based on Norwegian research. In: *Proceedings of the Third International Conference on Goat Production and Disease*, Scottsdale, Arizona, USA; Dairy Goat Journal Publishing Company, pp. 105–108.

Solaiman, S.G.; Qureshi, M.A.; Davis, G.; Sparks, J. (1988a) Induced copper toxicity in goats. (a) Toxicity. *Journal of Animal Science* **66**, Supplement 1, 371–372.

Solaiman, S.G.; Qureshi, M.A.; Sparks, J.; Davis, G. (1988b) Induced copper toxicity in goats. (b) Growth performance. *Journal of Animal Science* **66**, Supplement 1, 509.

Søli, N.E.; Frøslie, A. (1979) Copper, zinc and molybdenum in goat liver. *Acta Veterinaria Scandinavica* **20**, 45–50.

Søli, N.E.; Nafstad, I. (1978) Effects of daily oral administration of copper to goats. *Acta Veterinaria Scandinavica* **19**, 561–568.

Stapleton (1978) Cited in: Reis, P.J. (1982) Growth and characteristics of wool and hair. In: *Sheep and goat production*, Coop, I.E. (Ed.), Amsterdam, Netherlands, Elsevier.

Stohman *et al.* (1868) Cited in Haenlein, G.F.W. (1980b) Nutrient requirements of dairy goats – past and present. *International Goat and Sheep Research* **1**, 79–95.

Sutton, J.D.; Mowlem, A. (1989) A comparison of barley and molassed sugar beet feed for Saanen goats in early lactation. *Animal Production* **48**, 653.

Sykes, A.R.; Russel, A.J.F. (1991) Deficiencies of macro-elements in mineral metabolism. In: *Diseases of sheep*, 2nd Edition, Martin, W.B.; Aitken, I.D. (Eds), London, UK; Blackwell Scientific Publications, pp. 225–238.

Tan, C.M. (1988) Utilization of low quality roughages by goats and sheep. *Ph.D. Thesis, Lincoln College, University of Canterbury, New Zealand.*

Tan, C.M.; Poppi, D.P.; Sykes, A.R. (1987) Comparative aspects of rumen digestion in goats and sheep offered barley straw. In: *Proceedings 4th AAAP Animal Science Congress, New Zealand*, Reardon, T.F.; Adam, J.L.; Campbell, A.G.; Sumner, R.M.W. (Eds), p. 345.

Tanabe, S.; Kameoka, K. (1977) Growth and nutrient utilization by kids fed milk replacers containing isolated soybean protein as the sole source of protein. *Japanese Journal of Zootechnical Science* **48**, 361–370.

Taylor, C.R.; Shkolnik, A.; Dmi'el, R.; Baharav, D.; Borut, A. (1974) Running in cheetahs, gazelles and goats: energy cost and limb configuration. *American Journal of Physiology*, **227**, 848–850.

Teh, T.H.; Escobar, E.N.; Ivey, D.S.; Samms, C.A.; Sahlu, T. (1987) Effect of varying levels of salt on growth performance, digestibility and clinical responses of growing dairy goats. In: *Proceedings of the IV International Conference on Goats, Vol. 2*, Santana, O.P.; Silva, A.G. da; Foote, W.C. (Eds), Brasilia, Brazil; EMBRAPA-DDT, pp. 1543–1544.

Throckmorton, J.C.; Ffoulkes, D.; Leng, R.A.; Evans, J.V. (1982) Response to bypass protein and starch in Merino sheep and Angora goats. *Proceedings of the Australian Society of Animal Production* **14**, 661.

Treacher, T.T.; Mowlem, A.; Wilde, R.M.; Butler-Hogg, B. (1987) Growth, efficiency of conversion and carcass composition of castrate male Saanen and Saanen x Angora kids on a concentrate diet. *Annales de Zootechnie* **36**, 341–342.

Tyrrell, H.F.; Reid, J.T. (1965) Prediction of the energy value of cow's milk. *Journal of Dairy Science* **48**, 1215–1223.

Underwood, E.J. (1981) *The mineral nutrition of livestock.* 2nd Edition, Slough, UK; Commonwealth Agricultural Bureau.

Van Soest, P.J. (1982) *Nutritional ecology of the ruminant.* Corvallis, Oregon, USA; O and B Books Inc.

Vérité, R.; Michalet-Doreau, B.; Chapoutot, P.; Peyraud, J.L.; Poncet, C. (1987) *Bulletin Technique, C.R.Z.V. Theix,* **70**, 19–34.

Volker, L.; Steinberg, W. (1981) The vitamin requirements of goats – a review. In: *Nutrition and systems of goat feeding, Vol. 1,* Morand-Fehr, P.; Bourbouze, A.; Simiane, M. de (Eds), Paris, France; ITOVIC-INRA, pp. 226–231.

Wahed, R.A. (1984) A comparative study of roughage selection and utilisation by sheep and goats under stall-feeding conditions. *M.Phil. Thesis, University of Reading, UK.*

Wahed, R.A. (1987) Stall-feeding barley straw to goats: the effect of refusal-rate allowance on voluntary intake and selection. *Ph.D. Thesis, University of Reading, UK.*

Wahed, R.A.; Owen, E. (1986a) Comparison of sheep and goats under stall-feeding conditions: roughage intake and selection. *Animal Production* **42**, 89–95.

Wahed, R.A.; Owen, E. (1986b) The effect of amount offered on selection and intake of barley straw by goats. *Animal Production* **42**, 473.

Watson, C.; Norton, B.W. (1982) The utilization of pangola grass hay by sheep and Angora goats. *Proceedings of the Australian Society of Animal Production* **14**, 467–470.

Webster, A.J.F.; Kitcherside, M.A.; Kierby, J.R.; Hall, P.A. (1984) Evaluation of protein feeds for dairy cows. *Animal Production* **38**, 548, Abstract.

Wentzel, D.; Vosloo, L.P. (1975) Dimensional changes of follicles and fibres during pre- and postnatal development in the Angora goat. *Agroanimalia* **7**, 61–64.

Westhuysen, J.M. van der; Wentzel, D.; Grobler, M.C. (1985) *Angora goats and mohair in South Africa.* Port Elizabeth, South Africa; South African Mohair Growers Association.

Weston, R.H.; Cantle, J.A. (1982) Voluntary roughage consumption in growing and lactating sheep. *Proceedings of the Nutrition Society of Australia* **7**, 147.

Wilke, P.I.; Smith, A.; Clur, B. (1981) Intake and excretion of sodium and potassium by milch goats receiving sodium hydroxide treated roughage. In: *Nutrition and systems of goat feeding, Vol. 1,* Morand-Fehr, P.; Bourbouze, A.; Simiane, M. de (Eds), Paris, France; ITOVIC-INRA, pp. 218–225.

Wilkinson, J.M.; Stark, B.A. (1987a) The nutrition of goats. In: *Recent advances in animal nutrition 1987,* Haresign, W.; Cole, D.J.A. (Eds), London, UK; Butterworths, pp. 91–106.

Wilkinson, J.M.; Stark, B.A. (1987b) *Commercial goat production.* Oxford, UK; BSP Professional Books.

Williams, R.J. (1993a) An empirical model for the lactation curve of white British dairy goats. *Animal Production* **57**, 91–97.

Williams, R.J. (1993b) Influence of farm, parity, season and litter size on the lactation curve parameters of white British dairy goats. *Animal Production* **57**, 99–104.

Winter, J.; Gorsch, R. (1974) Ziegen als Versuchstiere – ein Beitrag zur Fütterungsoptimierung. *Zeitschrift für Versuchstierkunde* **16**, 256–265.

Wolter, R. (1988) Alimentation vitaminique. In: *Alimentation des bovins, ovins et caprins,* Jarrige, R. (Ed.), Paris, France; Institut National de la Recherche Agronomique, pp. 113–120.

Wood, J.D. (1984) Composition and eating quality of goats meat. In: *Developments in goat production, 1984,* Proceedings of the Inaugural Conference of the Goat Producers' Association of Great Britain, 17 April 1984.

Yan, T.; Cook, J.E.; Gibb, M.J.; Ivings, W.E.; Treacher, T.T. (1993) The effects of quantity and duration of milk feeding on the intake of concentrates and growth of castrated male Saanen kids to slaughter. *Animal Production* **56**, 327–332.

Index

Figures in **bold** indicate major references.
Figures in *italic* refer to diagrams, photographs and tables.

Printed and bound by CPI Group (UK) Ltd, Croydon, CR0 4YY

12/01/2026

14805385-0001